Dr. Deah's

CALMANAC

YOUR INTERACTIVE MONTHLY GUIDE FOR CULTIVATING A POSITIVE BODY IMAGE

WRITTEN BY
DR. DEAH SCHWARTZ
ED.D, CTRS, CCC

Illustrations By
BRENDA BROWN

Cover and book design by Ross Turner
ROSSTURNERDESIGN.COM

Cover illustrations and book illustrations by Brenda Brown
WEBTOON.COM

Printed in the United States of America

First Printing: December 2013
Dr. Deah's Body Shop: Book Division

ISBN 978-0-9912353-0-8

Contents

THIS WORK OF LOVE IS
DEDICATED TO YOU
AND YOUR ONGOING WORK OF
LOVING YOURSELF

WHY I WROTE THIS BOOK

A Tale of Two Cities

Let's play a game.

I say, "East Oakland, California."

You say, "__________."

Before I moved here in 1989, I called the local police and checked in about the crime stats. After all, I would most likely be raising a family at some point and wanted to hedge my bets proactively. I was told that the neighborhood was, "relatively safe with an occasional drive by."

With that knowledge tucked under my belt, contracts were signed and I moved in. Two weeks later, the Loma Prieta earthquake hit and my tiny little one story house, nonplussed, emerged safe and sound. It was like the airplane scene from *The World According to Garp*. Robin Williams, who plays the part of Garp, is looking at a home to purchase and an airplane flies into the house and bursts into flames. Garp looks at the realtor and says, "I'll take the house, what else could happen?"

I have lived here ever since.

–

The crime in my neighborhood has had its ups and downs over the years with the increases in crime seemingly in sync with economic downturns and desperation. I've been robbed once and on another occasion had a SWAT team (no, I'm not exaggerating or using poetic metaphor) in my back yard. But I still "hella love" Oakland.

One of the gems of this iconoclastic city by The Bay, and especially close to my heart, is Lake Merritt. The Lake is a remarkable place of refuge in the midst of a city known for its turmoil. It is a bird sanctuary, children's playground, nature and science learning center and the walking, biking and running tracks for many an Oaklander. I joined that "team" of Lake Walkers in 2002 after a serious back injury and have been walking the 3.4 mile circuit almost daily in order to stave off the immobilizing back spasms.

I always walk in the same direction which means that I have, over the years, met about a dozen or so people who are "walking The Lake" at the same time as I but in the opposite direction. It's amazing how hand waves and one- to three-word exchanges each day over the course of ten years weaves relationships with people whose names I don't even know.

But it does. When one of my "regulars" disappeared for a few months, my head was filled with questions about what happened to him… Was he okay? Had he moved, or merely changed direction? When I saw him one morning back in his regular spot, I waved, "Are you okay? I was worried about you!" He smiled and we high-fived each other. Over the course of the week, as we walked past each other, I learned of his close encounter with a stroke and gradual recovery. Goosebumps ran up and down my spine as I realized that he and I are as much a part of the ecosystem there as the pelicans, cormorants and grebes who have their own special sections of The Lake as they come and go with migration patterns as predictable as our daily walks.

–

But one day, things changed. I was the victim of a drive-by shouting.

No, it wasn't the first in my lifetime, but it was the first time at The Lake and it cut through me like a scalpel.

I was happily walking my route, savoring the sun and grateful for the crisp breeze against my face. As a transplanted New Yawker, I still get a satisfied feeling each December when I can leave my house without a snow shovel and in a T-shirt. I had just passed one of my favorite regulars, a young man in his late 20s who sports a pony tail and a black suit. Not a running suit, mind you, but a full-on matching set of black pants and button down jacket. It took about a year before I could elicit a brief two-finger forehead salute from him and another year before the wave was accompanied by a smile. Today he actually said, "Hi!" and I was filled with a sense of satisfied connection. Suddenly a car going in the opposite direction sped by, and in an instant my content became contempt.

The driver aimed and fired:

Walk it off, Baby, walk it off!

And he was gone.

Gone before I could respond. Gone before I could recover. Gone. Gone. Gone.

I was left fuming, stewing, hurting. Now, please trust me that I do NOT take violent crime lightly nor do I think that a drive-by shooting and a drive-by shouting are the same. I know they are not. But if you would indulge me and work with my metaphor, you'll understand why this type of "assault" is such a big deal to me. His words eclipsed any and all feelings of pleasure that I had been experiencing. I began to spiral down into a very bad case of the "should haves". As I trudged along, I went through a mental Rolodex of: "I should have said this," "I should have said that." "If I had his license plate number I'd find him and tell him this or that." My imagination on fire, I was in Dr. Deah's Hollywood.

Hello officer, I'd like to report a drive by shouting.

You mean shooting?

Okay, yes… A drive by shooting off of a mouth.

Yes, there were injuries.

I even crossed into the territory of blaming the victim:

> *Deah, why are you so sensitive? Why can't you just let these things roll off your shoulders? Why give him so much power?*

I also considered his point of view… perhaps he felt he was helping. Maybe he imagined himself a male Jillian Michaels on wheels and was convinced he was shouting out supportive, coach-like positive reinforcement because, after all, wouldn't the only reason that I'd be out there power walking around The Lake be to walk off my big ol' booty?

But in the end I kept coming back to the anger. If I saw him again I'd be prepared. I'd head him off at the stop sign. I'd lean in toward the car. I would aim and fire,

> *Did I ask for your help??? What you said didn't help. I don't want your help! Your help is based on assumptions and a one-sided point of view. How dare you intrude into my world only to wound me with your misguided bullets of support. The only thing I have to walk off, Babeee, is the anger, hurt, and humiliation you left in your so-called "helpful" wake.*

Sigh. As if…

As a person who has devoted decades to repairing wounds inflicted by "good intentions," it is startling to find that I am still vulnerable when I am the target of an emotional drive by. But I am human, and hence, an on-going work in progress. For a few days after the incident I noticed that I was more hyper-vigilant. There was less of a jaunt in my step, and I felt vulnerable. I wondered if everyone assumed that my walking regimen was motivated by my need to fit in to what society expects a woman's body to look like.

I thought of T-shirts I could wear.

> *Don't Help!*

Or,

> *I am Walking 4 my Health: NOT 2 B a Size 4*

Or,

> *Who Asked U?*

Or,

> *Occupy my Big Fat…*

Well, you get the idea…The good news is that my recovery time is quicker than it used to be, and I no longer punish myself for not being perfect in the eyes of others. The inner "should have" voices are quiet again and the PTSD (Post-Traumatic Shouting Damage) symptoms have faded. I'm back at The Lake walking and reveling in all she has to offer, geese and all!

The Lake is home for many Canadian geese. Not everyone loves the geese. They can be noisy, intrusive, and function as living movable speed bumps for the humans trying to make good time in their runs. There is also the issue of copious amounts of goose guano, which provides an organic obstacle course for those trying to maintain the pristine condition of their footwear. I tend to enjoy the geese, along with the other birds, but even I have been known to occasionally mutter frustrated warnings of "foie gras!" and "pâté!" when they block my way or hiss at me as I trudge up one of the few steep grades in the three-mile walk.

More typically, however (no offense to the geese) I take them in as part of the milieu and don't pay much attention to them.

Yesterday was different.

"GOOOOOOOSE!"

The delighted squeal of a child screamed out and pierced through my reverie forcing me to take a gander to see who was so excited about something so common place to the jaded joggers and weary walkers. I looked around and spotted the source. There was a little kid with itsy-bitsy corn rows, maybe three or four years old, pointing at a gaggle of geese and enthusiastically screaming:

"Look Mom, Look at that goose!"

Mom: "Uh-huh."

"That goose is so fat!"

Mom: "Uh-huh."

"It's a Big Fat Goose, Mom!"

Mom: "Uh-huh, yes it is."

"It's the fattest goose in the yard!"

Mom: "Yes, it is a very fat goose."

And then something shinier must have caught his attention and the goose was forgotten and the moment was over – for him.

It lingered for me.

As I resumed walking, I realized that I had been holding my breath and had stopped in my tracks to eavesdrop on the conversation. I noticed that my hands were clenched; in fact, my whole body was tense. As my hands and stomach began to relax and my breathing returned to normal, it dawned on me that I had shifted into a defensive state of mind, waiting for what I thought would be the inevitable additional adjectives that would most certainly follow.

Big, fat, ugly, goose. Big, fat, stupid, goose. Big, fat, yucky, goose.

But it never happened.

Here was someone who, despite his age, properly used the word fat as an adjective. Just an adjective. And it was a beautiful thing.

As I walked on, I wondered what his mom had been thinking during the exchange. I was curious if she had specifically role modeled any non-judgmental language usage or if he was just too young to have been exposed to the countless media messages telling him that fat was bad and that fat people were stupid, lazy, ugly, etc.? I pondered over whether it would have been different if he was commenting on a person instead of a goose?

I have lived a lifetime of being called fat, and NEVER has it been used to simply describe the parts of my body that were fat. And like any negative stereotyping, the labeling is accompanied by an attitude of disgust, pity, judgment, and coupled with assumptions about my personality and character. I laughed at myself as I realized that I was actually jealous of the goose for not having been attacked for the size of its body. I envied the fact that the goose was actually being admired for its size!

I am not sure how long this wee imp of a kid will be able to hold on to his non-judgmental perception of fat or whether someday it will be okay for geese to be fat but not people; but in that one moment around The Lake, I got a peek of what it could be like. What it should be like. What it would be like if negative messages about fat people were not accepted and common place everywhere we go.

The deleterious effects of weight stigma are indisputable, and quite frankly, avoidable.

Back in Dr. Deah's Hollywood, this story about walkers and geese goes viral and finds its way to the drive-by shouters. In a cinematic montage we see the people who believe they are doing a good deed, through their unsolicited coaching and commenting, having an epiphany. In a classic "light bulbs flashing" scene we witness "AHA!" moments, one after another:

> *– I get it… She isn't a project that needs fixing.*
>
> *– Eureka! She has her own valid definition of beauty!*
>
> *– What is that you say? A health-focused approach to living life and NOT a weight-focused approach?*
>
> *– Oh! It's none of my fracking business and I should keep my mouth shut!*
>
> *–Hmmm, maybe what's good for the goose is good for…*

We see them drive by grinning and nodding their heads and not disrupting The Lake's placid ecosystem. Change is in the air and all body self-consciousness has evaporated; geese waddle by and we fade to black.

But until then, here in Dr. Deah's Oakland, when I walk, I wear my Association of Size Diversity and Health (ASDAH) "Leave No Body Behind" T-shirt. And if anyone asks me how I feel about The Lake my answer will be, "It's a great neighborhood, relatively safe, with the occasional drive by."

> *Body dissatisfaction, disordered eating patterns, a preoccupation with physical appearance among girls has increased dramatically since the 1980s with 70-80% of fourth grade girls in the United States reporting they would rather be dead than fat.*

When I wrote this statement in 2001 for my doctoral dissertation about Body Image in Girls, and then re-used it in my first book, *Leftovers, the Workbook*, in 2008, I hoped that by 2013 the trend of increasing eating disorders, body hate, and size discrimination would have reversed. Sadly, the numbers have increased, crossed gender lines, and are more prevalent in boys and men than previously reported.

What has also grown is the body of research supporting that three primary factors predicting the onset of an eating disorder are body dissatisfaction (the judgmental feeling or perspective one has about their body), impaired body image (the inability to accurately judge the size of one's body), and societal and media influences (the obvious or hidden literary and visual messages that dictate what a person needs to look like in order to be considered beautiful or successful). Now, with the increased panic related to the perceived obesity epidemic, there is more pressure than ever for children and adults to conform to a narrow standard of body type – not just for beauty, but for health. The result, more people are being taught to hate their bodies. This, in turn, sets them on a course of self-loathing that negatively impacts their lives socially, emotionally, and sometimes vocationally.

The good news is there are more researchers, clinicians, organizations, and activists getting involved in providing the scientific data that reinforce the fact that diets don't work, most weight loss surgeries don't have the desired outcomes, and fat is not the enemy everyone has been taught to fear. In my line of work, the most important factor is that hating yourself is not good for your mental health. Hating your body is toxic and it is time for us to put the "heal" back in "health" and the "care" back in "healthcare."

This book is written with those goals in mind.

Less is Not More

Recently I purchased a box of Cheerios. This was not typical for me. Historically, I have never been a big Cheerios fan. But this was no ordinary box of Cheerios. This was "New Multi-Grain Peanut Butter" Cheerios, and because historically I HAVE been a big peanut butter fan, I was curious how much peanut butter taste would make its way into the cereal bowl experience. Considering past promises of s'mores, Oreos, and chocolate chip cookie cereals never quite living up to the claim that I would be eating a healthy breakfast in the guise of a guilty pleasure – I was up for the adventure with spoon in hand – albeit ready to be disappointed. So it was no surprise that as I sampled my first taste I was hit with the reality that I was eating a spoonful of mediocre cereal and not a spoonful of crunchy peanut butter. What I was not prepared for was what came next. As I sat there eating my O's and reading the back of the box (okay, not exactly mindful eating, but who DOESN'T read the box when they eat cereal?) the following words jumped out at me: **"More grains. Less you!"** I put my spoon down, shifted into my mindful reading mode, and continued to examine the box more thoroughly.

"People who choose more whole grains tend to weigh less than those who don't."

"Whole grain as a part of a sensible diet can help you manage your weight."

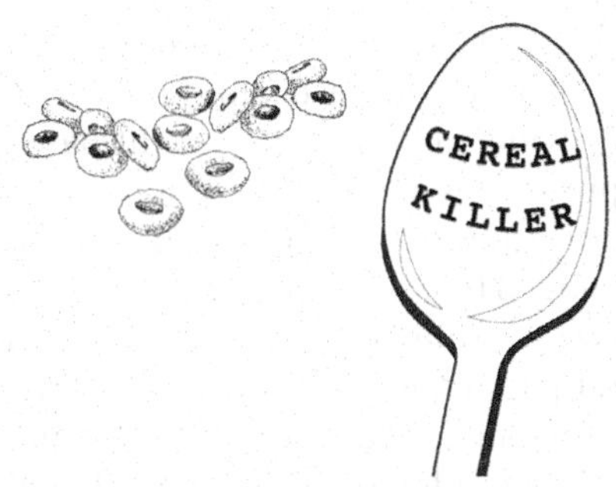

And just in case I missed it, there on the front of the box I was reminded,

"More grains. Less you!"

I felt my blood begin to boil as the wheels in my mind churned to comprehend what this box of cereal was saying to me. After decades of therapy working on self-acceptance and developing a healthy body image, I was being told that the world would be better off if there was less of me.

After years of learning how to, without apology, "own my space" and use my voice sans worry of coming off too opinionated or too large of a woman, this cereal box was telling me that my life would be better if there was less of me.

But what if I don't want to be less me? What if I am fine with "the me" that I am?

My-grain was rapidly transforming into a mi-graine as my train of thought increased speed. I told myself that perhaps I was being too picky and too literal; but think of it: Cheerios is telling women (and it is focused on women; the quotes and illustration on the box are all from a woman's perspective) that there is too much of us and we would be better off if there was less of us. The main reason for eating this cereal is to diminish our size.

Words are very important to me, but I know that not everyone scrutinizes the English language the way I do. Hence, I am curious if anyone else experienced cognitive dissonance from eating cereal for nutrition, flavor, and to satisfy hunger while concurrently being fed the message that consuming this food will result in less of you to nourish?

And what about people who feel they have nothing to lose or who are trying to increase their weight? Do they walk away from the chance to eat this presumably scrumptious promise of a bowl of peanut butter oats because they can't afford to be any less than what they already are?

The sociological undertones are also troubling. When a segment of the population, in this case overweight people, are being told that they are not okay unless there is less of them – well, you don't have to stretch that metaphor much to understand just how offensive the message is.

Fortunately, I was not the first person to complain about Multi-Grain Peanut Butter Cheerios. It turns out that there was parental outrage on behalf of children with peanut allergies in January, 2012, when the cereal was first introduced. Written about in the *Washington Post* and

SF Gate newspapers, parents voiced their concern about cross contamination between the peanut and non-peanut Cheerios. One of their complaints was that the box looked too similar to regular Cheerios, resulting in mistakenly purchasing the peanut O's. They asked that changes be made.

I wondered what would happen if parents of children with eating disorders took a page from the book of the national organization Allergy Moms, and lodged complaints with General Mills about the offensive slogans. Here's my thinking:

Part of establishing a healthy relationship with food is fostering the ability to eat foods based on internal cues and focus on satiety, hunger and appetite as reasons for eating. We already know that restrictive dieting and body dissatisfaction are contributing factors to eating disorders, and that focusing on a health-based style of living in lieu of a weight-based approach is an efficacious way to recover from body hate and disordered eating. Here is a product that has based its entire insulting ad campaign and packaging on promoting restrictive dieting, negative body image, and adds the additional component that you can "cheat" and eat one of the most formidable forbidden foods – peanut butter – and still lose weight.

For me the choice was simple. I wrote a letter to General Mills. But what worries me is the insidious way this product promotes body hate and reinforces the belief that the best me is less me.

I just don't and won't buy it.

Dr. Deah's CALMANAC

A 12-Month Guide for Cultivating a POSITIVE BODY IMAGE

An almanac is an annual manual containing important dates, advice and information relating to a sport or pastime. *The Old Farmer's Almanac*, one of the most renowned examples of this genre, also includes salient information for growing and harvesting hearty and plentiful crops and gardens.

Almanacs are helpful for a variety of reasons, but in my book (literally and figuratively), it is the calming effect that I find most beneficial – hence the name "Dr. Deah's Calmanac". I know, I know; groan ... pun ... groan... But in the spirit of full disclosure, if you have a low tolerance for puns, you should return this book immediately for a full refund (minus the shipping) – this Calmanac is rife with puns because I believe that humor is a wonderful thing. But why do I find almanacs calming?

–

Living in this world is, for most of us, a combination of repetitive routines and hectic, unpredictable occurrences. Successfully navigating our day-to-day course usually means: having to accommodate for unexpected events and keeping track of daily responsibilities.

Not all unplanned events are negative. Along with the potholes and flat tires, we hopefully hear from an old friend or serendipitously meet a new one. But either way, adapting to this multifaceted terrain of life takes energy, focus, and finding a balance. Even the most resilient and flexible person can find themselves accruing tension and anxiety from trying to adjust to the fluctuations of daily life, and before we know it, stress has become a steady and unshakable traveling companion.

In the same way that each day can be both predictable and surprising, each month offers its own particular challenges for people struggling with body dissatisfaction or disordered eating. For some, this repetitive, cyclical nature of the seasons can tap into feelings of apathy and hopelessness: a sense of inevitability that nothing will change, nothing can change – or, paradoxically – that the constant pattern changes and fluctuations will never stabilize. But remember, our history is not fate – it is knowledge, and our past does not dictate our present or future behaviors. We can learn from our past, hold on to the positives, and choose to throw the negatives in the mulch bin. In order to reap the benefits of the repetition or redundancy that our calendar year presents, it is imperative that we take some time to examine the months and seasons for their predictable ebbs and flows. Then like any successful farmer, we can plan our garden of positive body image around the elements that are most certain to occur. This is sounding quite a bit almanacky to me! One of the outcomes of seeing the patterns and order in chaos is a sense of safety, control, and calmness.

Sow, Here's the Plan

Each chapter in this Calmanac is associated with a month of the year, and has four components:

Personal Perspective: My real-life musings on body image and disordered eating.

Predictable Challenges: Common themes to be aware of during the month.

Important Dates to Remember: Opportunities for activism or possible triggers that arise in that month.

Proactive Activities or "Proactivities": Two expressive arts directives that address the themes discussed in "Predictable Challenges."

These arts directives may be used by individuals or in a group. Sometimes, the activity itself is nothing new, but the objective of the directive is unique and specifically tailored to exploring issues related to body image and disordered eating. You will not find any photographs of sample finished pieces. I believe that comparisons can be stifling and inhibit the creative process. Hopefully the directions are written carefully enough that a visual aid will not be necessary. If you have a question about any of the steps in the Proactivities, please contact me and I will help clarify them for you.

–

Now, chances are, if this book has found its way into your hands, you are either related to me or curious about how to improve your or someone else's body image. It is my fervent desire that you, the reader, turn this book into your book. PLEASE PLEASE PLEASE do not feel obligated to actually do all of the Proactivities in this book. I hate it when people tell me what to do. I have piles of workbooks on my shelves where every worksheet is pristine and untouched. It doesn't mean I didn't reap any benefits from the book. *Dr. Deah's Calmanac* is not another diet book or weight loss program. I don't want this to be a new opportunity for you to feel like a failure if you don't feel like doing the projects. That being said, I encourage you to read through each one of them. Perhaps you will agree with me that by simply reading the "**How To**" and "**Why**" sections of each Proactivity, some seeds of thought about ways to grow a more positive body image will be planted.

If you do choose to do any or all of the Proactivities, try to set aside enough time so you don't feel rushed. It will be helpful to have a box of supplies already collected to use including: scissors, glue, paper of varying sizes, markers, pencils, and magazines. Try to limit the number of fashion magazines, they can be triggering. Most importantly remember, there is no right or wrong way to complete the Proactivities. Not that you need it, but you have my permission to add your own ingredients to the process. And, remember, fun and humor are always welcome.

Let's Get GROWING!

JANUARY
A New Year

Personal Perspectives

I have to make a confession.

I am not a big fan of New Year's Eve.

In fact, in the spirit of full disclosure, I hate New Year's Eve.

I hate it hate it hate it!!!!!

When I was little, I hated New Year's Eve because the grownups were clearly waiting for the kids to go to sleep so they could do something special. They put on their fancy clothes, set out special cocktail napkins, and, as the doorbell began to ring, the kids were sent to bed. I felt excluded and disappointed.

By the time I was allowed to stay up until midnight, the thrill had mysteriously faded for my parents. They weren't dressing up in their fancy clothes, there were no cocktail napkins laid out, and I could tell they were counting the minutes until the clock struck 12:00 so they could go to sleep. I remember one year in particular when they actually went to bed before the ball dropped. Still searching for the magic of the New Year's Eve moment, I went into the basement with my cat and at the strike of 12:00 I blew a horn and threw confetti up in the air. As I swept up the confetti before I went to bed, I felt excluded and disappointed.

As a young adult, New Year's Eve took on a whole new significance as it became all about the midnight kiss. We gathered at a friend's house whose parents had gone out for the night. Dressed up in my fancy clothes, I furtively sipped champagne and hoped that a boy would be in close proximity as the ball dropped and he would kiss me as I entered the New Year. It was all about being chosen. No one kissed me. I felt excluded and disappointed.

Now, as an adult, firmly planted in my 50s, I watch others revel and drunkenly clink glasses while waiting for the ball to drop. I listen to the chorus of "Happy New Year" and am surprised to find the old feelings of disappointment and alienation filling my belly. Why do I feel this way? I am no longer excluded from the festivities, I am of legal drinking age, and I have a wonderful someone to kiss me at the stroke of midnight.

I think part of it is the hypocrisy that is associated with New Year's Eve. I hate that everyone says "Happy New Year," when in reality most everyone is focused on what is NOT happy about their lives, hence the self-flagellating tradition of New Year's resolutions.

Happy New Year!

As the ball drops, people find comfort in knowing they are part of a community of people who have made New Year's resolutions. There is hope and a sense of inclusion – and yet, more often than not, the resolutions are unrealistic. It won't be long before they drop the ball of implementing those impossible promises and are, perhaps, left feeling… excluded and disappointed.

Where is the "happy" in focusing on our failures and weaknesses? Where is the "happy" in a collective consciousness of "I am a loser"? Where is the "happy" in only acknowledging what <u>didn't</u> work last year and setting unattainable goals for what will make the next year happier than last year was? And where is the "new" or the "happy" about people selling products that capitalize on our despondency or desperate annual pursuit of perfection?

Please don't misinterpret me. I'm not saying it's a bad idea to have goals or objectives for changing our lives for the better. Nor am I saying there is no room for self-improvement; most of us can find ways to take better care of ourselves. **I need to floss more. I know it, my dentist knows it, and now you know it.**

But what I am objecting to is the oppressive and negative nature of the New Year's resolution mind set.

I understand the temptation to use the calendar to define beginnings and endings. It's part of our culture, after all, to use birthdays and anniversaries as structural tools. So it makes sense to use a momentous date like the first day of the New Year to put a new foot forward, so to speak. But <u>what if</u> we started from a more positive place and focused on what worked well during the previous year and identified things we want to continue to do or expand upon because they worked?

Or...

<u>What if</u> we chose resolutions that were less punitive and more attainable; or got really crazy and resolved to do a few things to make another person's life better? My hunch is that, with a few of those types of adjustments to the resolution ritual, there would be less money lining the pockets of the Jenny Craigs of the world and fewer depressed people in March when the hopefulness surrounding the unattainable resolution has predictably waned. I think the current system is broken and wouldn't be that difficult to resolve.

If you do feel compelled to make a resolution, here are a few tips (feel free to add your own suggestions!):

• Steer clear of all-or-nothing goals. Remember that there is a middle ground in making behavioral and attitudinal changes:

• Start small. You can always increase your goal later on.... No, you don't have to wait until next December 31st to set a new goal.

• Choose measurable goals and objectives with positive reinforcements along the way.

• Create resolutions that are health focused and not weight focused.

• Co-resolute (I just made up that word) with a friend or a group. This lessens the chance of feeling disappointed or excluded. (Okay, maybe I'm projecting my own personal issues in this one).

• Remember what is wonderful and amazing about you and resolve to acknowledge and appreciate yourself!

• Floss! ;-)

Predictable Challenges

January 1st. It is day 1 of the NEW YEAR and purportedly filled with potential for so many people. We are bombarded by messages from the media, friends, family, co-workers, et cetera, that January is the month of resolutions. "I resolve to do this; I resolve not to do that." If you look at the words "resolution" and "resolve," they have a repetitive, cyclical feel to them. A resolution or to resolve gives the impression that it is time to try – yet again – to solve an old problem, pattern, or area of dissatisfaction. True, there can be more than one solution to a problem or at least more than one way to arrive at a solution, so exploring different avenues for problem solving is not necessarily a negative course; but frequently, when it comes to body image issues and eating disorders, New Year's resolutions tend to originate from self-hate and are all-or-nothing propositions:

I will stop eating anything after 6:00p.m. I will go to the gym EVERY day.

This "clean slate" mentality that accompanies New Year's resolutions is fertile ground for planting seeds of unattainable goals and unrealistic aspirations of perfection. For many of us grappling with body dissatisfaction, the flip side of setting New Year's resolutions is the dark underbelly of feeling like a failure and perseverating on what was wrong with us the previous year. This emphasis on not feeling capable of change and a heightened awareness of the repetitive nature of the years going by without making perceptible progress in certain areas of our lives may leave many of us feeling depressed and despondent. While it is tempting to use the first of the year as a jumping-off point to fix all that ails us, let's remember that each year is comprised of 365 days. Each of these days is an opportunity for improving our health and well-being by setting goals that are attainable and not weight based.

I am not saying that this is easy and will happen overnight. You will be swimming upstream against the tide once you decide to eschew the pressure of reinventing yourself on January 1st. Your decision appears even more rebellious and revolutionary to others if you choose to focus on the previous positive events that are worthy of celebration in the here and now. Perhaps cloaking your decision by using the standard lingo would be helpful:

> *I resolve not to make any resolutions that are outcroppings of self-hate.*

Did you know there are definitions for the word "resolution" that offer perspectives other than committing to a course of change in order to gratify our or someone else's opinion about what would make us more acceptable? For example, in physics or chemistry, resolution is the act of breaking something down into its components – e.g., looking at a rainbow and finding its individual colors. In the visual arts, resolution is how clear an image is on a computer screen or in a photograph. And in music, resolution is the process of changing a dissonant tone or chord to a consonant tone or chord.

People in Western cultures typically experience consonant chords as harmonious, while dissonant chords tend to elicit feelings of tension. When a composer moves from dissonant to consonant, the tension is released, and this is called resolution. But some composers may choose not to resolve the tension; they see no need to "fix" the piece or make it "right." They feel it adds variety and depth to a composition, and perhaps most importantly, they believe that experiencing musical dissonance as negative is a subjective and cultural preference that needs no resolution.

Imagine
LOOKING AT YOUR BODY AND FEELING NO NEED TO
"FIX IT"
OR MAKE IT
"RIGHT"

When it comes to body image – similar to music – our culture may dictate what is dissonant about our bodies and what needs resolution. We are taught what is harmonious about how we look and feel about our bodies and what causes dissatisfaction so extreme that a resolution to fix it takes center stage, at any price. There is a great deal of media, family, and peer pressure this time of year to make resolutions, and these expectations may be wrapped in layers of love, caring, and concern for our health. But what if we looked at the physics, chemistry, music, and visual arts concepts of resolution? By looking at ourselves and our lives through those lenses we can choose to:

- Reflect on our past and acknowledge what individual components are beneficial in our lives.
- Define our own goals of self-worth and self-acceptance instead of integrating other's perceptions as our own.
- Ascertain if there are aspects of our lives that we choose to adjust or fine tune in order to improve our quality of life.
- Discover the unique balance of consonance and dissonance about our bodies and our relationship with food.
- Fertilize and nurture our self-acceptance.
- Learn to love our bodies for their brilliance and ability to carry us through each day.

Important Dates to Remember

January offers two opportunities to test drive your new "resolution vehicle." Every January we honor Martin Luther King, a man of great resolve who believed in peaceful resolutions, and who preached the value of looking at our past and holding onto some of the traditional values in order to move forward and make progress. King never said it was easy to generate self-respect, internally or externally, but he was resolved to change cultural definitions of consonance and dissonance.

The third week of January in the U.S. is Healthy Weight Week (the fourth week in Australia), which provides us with numerous ways to choose body love over body hate and exposes the truth behind media-supported "quick fixes" that promise to resolve whatever dissonance we are holding in our bodies:

> *During Healthy Weight Week, people are encouraged to improve health habits in lasting ways and normalize their lives by eating well without dieting, living active lives, and accepting the notion of size diversity. Our bodies cannot be shaped at will. But we can all be accepting, healthy and happy at our natural weights.*
>
> -FRANCIE BERG

Francie M. Berg, a licensed nutritionist, has chaired Healthy Weight Week since 1992. Berg has this to say:

> *More people today know the value of size acceptance. They've experienced the harmful effects of dieting, idealizing thin models and harassing large children and adults. They're ready to move on.*

For more information on Healthy Weight Week you can visit healthyweight.net.

January 1 – New Year's Day
Third Monday of January – Martin Luther King Day
Third week of January – Healthy Weight Week

Proactivity # 1

Advent(ure) Calendars (A new spin on the advent calendar)

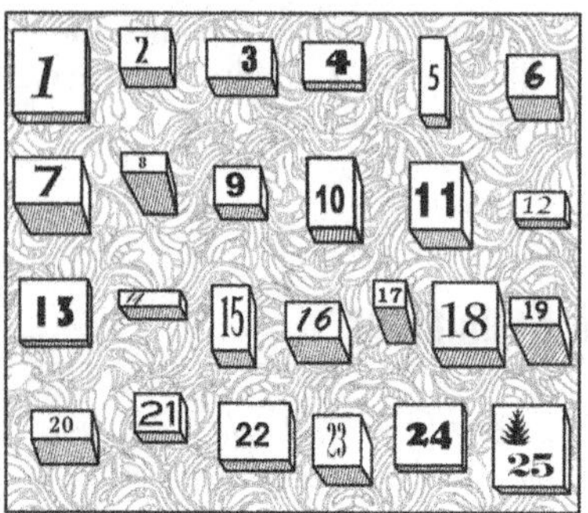

Materials

Poster board, manila file folders, card stock paper, ruler, scissors, markers, stickers, magazines, glue sticks, fabric, felt, paper bags, envelopes, yarn or magnetic strip for hanging, creativity, and imagination. Optional: Photos or samples of advent calendars.

–

How To

1. Brainstorm on small attainable goals that focus on improving self-esteem, healthy lifestyle, and/or helping someone else. These goals can be as simple as saying, "I am willing to learn something new today." Or inviting a friend to take a walk, or, "If I say or think something negative about myself I will say or think one positive thing about myself afterward." Try to have fun with this, get silly, get serious, and get ADVENTurous!

2. Try to come up with 31 ideas, but if that proves to be too difficult, come up with seven and reuse the ideas each week throughout the month.

3. Using the poster board or fabric, design a calendar grid. It doesn't have to be a standard looking grid. It can be different shapes and sizes for each day (see illustration).

4. Write down each goal/activity on a small piece of paper and fold in half.

5. Using a combination of felt, paper bags, envelopes, and paper, create a container or pouch for each note and attach one to each day on the grid.

6. Make one extra pouch and place somewhere on the calendar.

7. Randomly place one note inside each pouch.

8. Create a hanger with yarn or magnetic strip.

9. Each day, pull out the note and follow the plan to the best of your ability. When a goal is achieved, put the note back in the pouch. If a goal is not attained, place it in the extra pouch. At the end of the month you can see which goals you may want to try again the next month, and or explore what made those goals more difficult than the ones that were achieved.

–

Why

For those of you unfamiliar with advent calendars they are a unique calendar with flaps used to count or celebrate the days in anticipation of Christmas. Each day a flap is opened and a picture is revealed underneath. Making an advent calendar is not a new art activity, but rarely is it used as a delightful tool for charting progress and setting goals for improving body image. Since January is the month of New Year's resolutions, oftentimes people set unattainable long-term goals without measurable objectives and opportunities for positive reinforcement along the way. Setting an ambiguous goal, e.g., "I'll start going to the gym," "I'll lose weight," "I will exercise," gives few opportunities to feel good about progress. This Advent(ure) Calendar is set up for daily achievable goals tailored to increase self-esteem and adopt healthy habits that are not weight based. At the end of the month, there is tangible proof of what actions were taken towards improving quality of life (replaced in their pouch) and which were not (those in the extra pouch). Unlike most New Year's resolutions, this will last and stay pertinent month after month after month!

Notes

Notes

Proactivity # 2

Make Your Own Kind of Music

"You've got to make your own kind of music, sing your own special song. Make your own kind of music, even if nobody else sings along."

– "MAMA" CASS ELLIOT, VOCALIST

Materials

Any combination of collage materials, pens, pencils, paints, scissors, glue sticks, adhesive tape, and photographs: but be sure to have large sheets of paper for the foundation of the finished product. **Optional, but really fun:** An old vinyl album jacket or plastic CD case.

–

How To

1. On a piece of paper, without editing, write down aspects of yourself that you like and accept. These can be physical attributes, or skills, talents, frames of intelligence, etc.

2. Put a star next to items that you may like and accept about yourself even if other people don't.

3. Examine the list for any patterns of what you find acceptable about yourself. Make notes about any messages you received (and where they came from) about what was acceptable and what wasn't.

4. Now imagine you are designing an album or CD cover and using the available art materials create a visual representation of at least one aspect of yourself that you appreciate despite external pressure that you are wrong to feel this way. Are there symbols that illustrate what gives you the ability to do this? If you are using the jewel case or album cover, be sure the artwork fits on those surfaces.

5. If you want, you can continue the work on the flip side of the CD case or album cover. One variation is to list names of some of the songs you would include on the CD – either already-existing music or names you invent that pertain to the theme of self-acceptance – and "making your own kind of music."

6. Give the record/CD a title that represents the positive attribute you are acknowledging. Remember, we are identifying parts of us that we can hold onto in a positive, self-accepting way, despite what others may tell us, and this strength can be generalized to how we feel about our bodies.

–

Why

The purpose of this activity is to begin to explore our own definition of what is consonant and dissonant about our self-image. In Western culture, most of us are trained to feel tension when we hear dissonant chords and to feel harmony or release when the chord or tone is consonant. But our responses to music are subjective, and each one of us has our own unique preference as to what music we enjoy and how sound combinations make us feel.

Our culture has also influenced our opinion of our bodies and how we feel about ourselves. This activity is designed to help separate or identify sources of our negative body image and begin to define our own sense of body acceptance.

Notes

FEBRUARY
Mixed Nuts

Personal Perspectives

That's how I feel about Valentine's Day – like a can of mixed nuts.

In my home, when I was growing up, those cans of Planter's Mixed Nuts would magically appear once or twice a year in the living room. At first glance, they looked like the regular dark blue can of roasted salted peanuts with the iconic Mr. Peanut in top hat and monocle waving at me. Those were easy for me to ignore – peanuts were never my "fave." Why I love peanut butter but can live in the same house with a can of roasted salted peanuts without any temptation for noshing on them still mystifies me.

But this can, upon closer inspection, was the bonus can of "Mixed Nuts." If I was lucky to get to the can before my dad, there may have been some filberts left. I LOVED the filberts. If I got there before my sister, I could still score some pecans. But the true treasures for me were the cashews. Even rarer was finding a cashew in its entirety and not just a chip of the crescent or a split half. The mother lode for me was the full cashew.

I believe my earliest experience in mindful eating came the first time I ate a cashew. It was the perfect combination of salt, crunch, flavor, and texture: sweet and salty at the same time … and rich with a smoothness of oily crunchy goodness. YUM. But mostly, the can of mixed nuts was stuffed with peanuts, and someone else always seemed to get the cashews, and I was left feeling empty, left out, and craving something I couldn't quite put my finger on.

VALENTINES DAY
OVER THE YEARS
HAS MEANT
MANY THINGS
TO ME.

As a preschooler: It was an art project that my mom and I did together: cutting out lacy doilies and scribbling over the textured paper with red waxy crayons to see what shapes came out on the white paper beneath it. Then my mom would do the most amazing thing. She would fold the piece of paper in half, take the scissors, and execute some cuts. And when she was finished, she would reveal a heart filled with my scribbles. I couldn't understand how she could cut a piece of paper and still have it come out as a full piece and not split in half.

Valentine's Day was about miracles with my mom, and it was indeed a cashew.

As a girl in grammar school: Valentine's Day was about bringing valentines to your teacher and every kid in your class. The first year I remember diligently cutting out valentine after valentine – my mom having taught me the scissor trick by then – and bringing them into school eager to hand them out. To my horror, everyone else had brought in store-bought Snow White or Sleeping Beauty valentines, glittery, each in their own perfect tiny envelope, except the one for the teacher, which was much larger.

My valentines were the "peanuts," and I left school that day feeling empty, left out … and craving something I couldn't quite put my finger on.

As a preteen in junior high: While the tradition continued to bring in the mass-marketed valentines continued, now available in super heroes, Barbie, and Charlie Brown (literally *Peanuts* versions), what was written on the back of the valentine was the true valentine. Most of them were just "peanuts" signed by the person who, like me, had used the class list and written name after name on each card so as not to leave anyone out or hurt someone's feelings. But once in a while, you would get a note on the back that was different:

To the prettiest girl in homeroom.
Love, Gary

Wow … that was a cashew, a filbert, and pecan all rolled up in one!!!

As a young adult: Valentine's Day transformed into the day to express true love, romantic love – intimate, sexy, hot, passionate love. And, of course, if that was not in your life, it became the day of regrets and lamentations: Why am I alone? Why don't I have a valentine? Where is my Gary now? Then…If I were thinner, I'd have a Valentine. And I would think this to myself as I mindlessly and angrily ate a piece of heart-shaped candy that was given out at the hospital where I worked,

This whole February 14th thing is just a Hallmark opportunity to sell cards and make money.

As a new mom: When my son was 3, he and I sat at the kitchen table dutifully making valentines for all of the kids in his preschool. Surrounded by doilies, red crayons, and construction paper, we scribbled, cut and pasted enough valentines for each and every kid in his group and of course made one larger card for his teacher. I showed him how to fold a piece of paper in half and cut it so it came out in ONE piece shaped like a heart. His eyes were wide with wonder and glee. We used glitter and stickers, and he made one extra for himself. I smiled when I saw that. It had never occurred to me to make a valentine for myself, but somehow it felt right.

When I dropped him off the next morning, all of the other kids were marching in with their arms full of valentines. Some were homemade, some store bought, I grinned. I left feeling somewhat … full … hopeful … and satiated … as if I had had my fill of cashews.

TODAY: Whether we like it or not, we are bombarded by the media's messages that this special day is about buying the right gift and being loved or lovable.

I say, it is about connection. And the most important connection we can make is with ourselves. No, this is not selfish, narcissistic, or arrogant. It is healthy. What I learned from my 3-year-old son – which is, in fact, a universal truth – is that the most important valentine we can receive is the one we give ourselves from a place of self-love. Only then can we open up to the love of others and be able to love others as well. It is hard to believe I finally learned that there really are enough cashews for everyone.

Predictable Challenges

February is a month of unique challenges in the field of eating disorders, health and wellness, body image, and size acceptance. With the holiday season now officially over, February provides the chance to settle back into normal routines, less hectic schedules, and a respite from food-related festivities that surround the winter holidays. What a relief, especially for those of us who struggle with weight-cycling diets and binge eating.

Predictably, it is also the time when many of last month's New Year's resolutions to diet, work out, and lose weight begin to dissolve and are replaced by feelings of panic, disappointment, and anxiety. Thus, what should be a time for feeling more relaxed and less pressured may leave some of us spiraling down into feelings of failure and self-contempt.

February also brings us Valentine's Day: a holiday with seemingly good intentions of expressing our love for each other. Yet, sadly, Valentine's Day often has the paradoxical effect of people feeling unloved and unlovable often because of a negative body image.

And then, of course, what is the number one, most common way of showing someone that we love them on Valentine's Day???

Candy!

Isn't it ironic that so many women feel unloved and unlovable because of their negative body image and disordered-eating behaviors, and then, we have this holiday that has chocolate and being loved completely intertwined?

The Dr. Deah Optimistic Pollyanna reframe of this situation is how fortunate we are to once again have the opportunity to practice:

- Loving our body in the here and now.
- Seeing food as an enjoyable experience and NOT the enemy.
- Remembering that mindful (and enjoyable) eating does not mean an all-or-nothing approach to food – i.e., now I'm starving myself, now I'm bingeing.
- Forgiving ourselves and knowing that a happier life is not measured by a scale.

And perhaps most important of all:

- The most meaningful valentine anyone can receive is the one we give ourselves.

Let's celebrate Valentine's Day by taking advantage of the opportunity it provides us to reinforce the practice of self-love by quieting our negative and critical internal voices. And please remember this important distinction: Self-love is not synonymous with narcissism or selfishness. It is not arrogant to love who we are for who we are. Rather, this was our natural state before we were exposed to the bombardment of negative messages that surround us in a culture that promotes one narrow standard of beauty for all.

Important Dates to Remember

February 2: Not Just for Groundhogs Anymore!!!

February 2nd is Groundhog Day. Before 1993, Groundhog Day was all about whether the infamous groundhog, Punxsutawney Phil, was going to pop out of his burrow and see his shadow or not. Everyone crossed their fingers, hoping that he would not see his shadow, because this indicated that winter would last for another six weeks, and then Phil would retreat to his underground home.

Personally, if I was Punxsutawney Phil and I popped up out of my burrow and saw throngs of strange people standing around staring at me, I'd pop back underground in a flash whether it meant six more weeks of winter or not! Now that I think of it, I can't remember a single time that Phil did NOT immediately retreat, and having grown up in New York, it sure never felt like winter ended early!

But then, in 1993, the movie *Groundhog Day* came out, and the phrase "Groundhog Day" took on a new meaning. If you are not familiar with the Bill Murray film, he is thrust into a reality where he keeps reliving Groundhog Day over and over and over. Each morning he wakes up and it is the same day; each day he knows what is going to happen and eventually begins using the predictability in ways that are helpful to others. He transforms into a more aware and less self-centered person as he plays with the hand that fate dealt him.

One of the meta-messages of the film is that, for all of us, in some ways, life is like *Groundhog Day*. Each morning when we wake up, we have a chance to pay closer attention to ourselves and to those around us. Every day we have a new opportunity to recalibrate our "personal frequency receivers" and tune into events that sometimes seem invisible to us because we are busy, distracted, or just unconsciously going through our daily routines.

We assume that things may be the same because they look the same, and we are not used to digging deeper. Yet, when we do dig deeper, the insights that result or knowledge we uncover can be invaluable for our personal journey to self-acceptance. And we can then help educate others as well.

This year on February 2, take a moment before popping out of bed, and consciously decide to be more attentive to yourself and your experience as you go through the day. Notice your patterns, your negative thought cycles, and how you handle positive feedback or thoughts:

- What are your interactions with others about your body and food?
- Are you engaging in negative body talk?
- Are you allowing yourself to appreciate your body for the wonderful miraculous things it accomplishes?

Give it a try. It's just one day! See what you discover.

And speaking of awareness, did you know that the fourth week of February is National Eating Disorders Awareness (NEDA) Week? According to NEDA, The aim of NEDA Awareness Week is to:

> *Ultimately prevent eating disorders and body image issues while reducing the stigma surrounding eating disorders and improving access to treatment. Eating disorders are serious, life-threatening illnesses – not choices – and it's important to recognize the pressures, attitudes and behaviors that shape the disorder.*

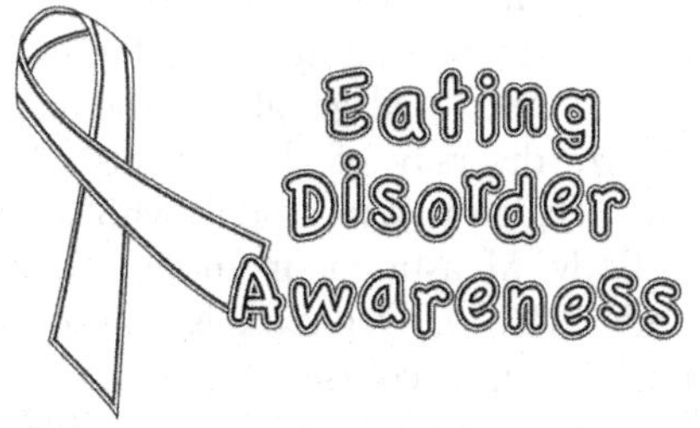

During this week, the goal is for everyone to do just one thing to help raise awareness and provide accurate information about eating disorders.

More information about NEDA Week can be found at: nedawareness.org

Fashion Week

I am not sure if this was intentional planning or just a coincidence, but February also brings us Fashion Week. So, at the same time that we are hopefully reading and sharing messages about the importance of preventing eating disorders and how the media's obsession with thinness is one of the primary causes of body dissatisfaction, we are also being kept up to date on the latest, trendiest fashions on the runway. The typical size of fashion models used during Fashion Week supports the paradigm that beauty comes in a one-size-fits-very-few wrapper. This can be mind boggling for those of us working on establishing our own definition of beauty and body positivity.

Every February, New York City hosts an international extravaganza of fashion. On the upside, there has been an increasing amount of public protest and outrage about the lack of size diversity of the models. Israel decided to ban models who have a Body Measurement Index (BMI) under 18.5%, Denmark is considering the same course of action, and fashion shows in Madrid and Milan have disallowed models on the runway with BMI's below 18 and 18.5% respectively, citing that a 5'8" model with a BMI of 18.5% would weigh about 119 pounds. Their belief is that sustaining that weight for many girls and women who are not genetically prone to be that size may demand disordered eating behaviors. People are hoping that these restrictions will curtail the increasing percentage of young women who suffer from eating disorders in order to become or emulate the fashion models. And the ultimate outrage: Did you know that scouts for fashion models frequently approach girls leaving clinics and doctor's offices that treat eating disorders?

Now, if I learned one thing in my Doctoral Statistics Classes (lovingly known as Sadistic Classes) it was that "correlation does not always mean causation." Simply put, just because it appears that something causes something it doesn't mean that it does. But it is difficult to ignore the growing body of research that connects the unrealistic and unattainable standards of beauty in fashion magazines with a marked increase of young girls developing eating disorders. So while the Fashion Industry may not actually be one of the causes of this increase in body dissatisfaction and eating disorders, perhaps it may be still be a positive step to have a variety of body types and sizes represented on the runway.

On the downside, despite the outcry of concern regarding using models with extremely low BMI's, Fashion

Week 2013 did not include a more diverse representation of bodies.

For many of us who grew up on the East Coast, another annual tradition in February is the *New York Times'* Special Fashion Magazine Section; an insert reporting the highlights of Fashion Week. This year was no exception, and it was predictably filled with photographs of redundantly identical-looking models clad in the creations of the major international fashion houses. As I thumbed through this big glossy publication looking and hoping for any exceptions to the rule, none were found.

I flashed back to my teenage years when I would go through this same ritual in my living room in New York, feeling desperate to grow six inches taller and lose fifty pounds so that I, too, could look like the women in the magazine. There was not one model that came close to resembling my short, curvy body, which meant I was destined to NEVER be fashionable EVER. It is amazing how tangible and painful those memories still feel decades later, and I wince when I think about all the years I suffered trying to conform. I don't always look at the magazine anymore, but this year I was optimistic. Maybe this was due to the Israeli decision coupled with the incremental changes I've seen in my work involving size/fat acceptance. I was curious to see if it was evident in a more mainstream publication. Mostly, though, it was because I had hoped that who I saw on the cover of the magazine was a harbinger of what I would find inside the February, 2013 issue.

In a milieu where the average age of models appears to be predominantly teens with a smattering of geriatrics in their early '20s, seeing the 79-year-old grand dame Lee Radziwill, sister of Jacqueline Kennedy-Onassis, unapologetically looking her age, was a delightful change. Yes, she was tall, rail thin, and hence labeled elegant, but perhaps this would be just one image of many inside the cover that challenged the stereotype of the fashion model having to be one age range and one size. It was a hope that dissipated rapidly.

R(age) Before Beauty

Back to the upside. (This is like the stock market!)

I lead workshops for women on body image, redefining beauty, and eating disorder prevention. A topic that emerges most every time is along with the pressure for women to be thin, is the demand to be young. Aging (the unavoidable result of not dying) is being sold as the enemy of beauty. And in a world that still views beauty and success as inseparable, being fat and older is a toxic cocktail guaranteeing a stock market crash of self-esteem.

The fashion, diet, and cosmetic industries, in pursuit of generating money, are now selling age-related self-hate with similar financial rewards as fat self-hate. Creams, lotions, diets, nutritional tips, "non-fail" exercise regimes, and, of course, surgery, all promise to reclaim and retain the youthful appearance women are desperate to hold onto.

But we have the right to fight back. What if we work together to change the paradigm and give ourselves and all women permission to celebrate the visible signs of a well-laughed, well-cried, and well-lived life? There are two organizations doing just that: Miss Representation and About Face (more about them can be found in the resource section) are running ardent campaigns challenging these ageist, size-ist, and sexist paradigms of what constitutes beauty and teaches us how to reduce the importance of beauty as a definition for success. There is valuable healing to be found by plugging into organizations that offer us a self-affirming message as opposed to a self-degrading one.

The self-acceptance journey that we are on is difficult. No one is saying it isn't. But it is a journey that is made easier with support and community – a community that celebrates and honors diversity and demands equal representation of all natural shapes, sizes, and ages.

February 2 – Groundhog Day
Fashion Week New York City – varies
Third Monday in February – President's Day
Fourth week in February – NEDA week

Proactivity # 1

Expressive He(art)s

Materials

White paper, pencils, gloves (no need to be matched pairs). Wool or cotton is preferable, but rubber or latex gloves are fine as well. (Be careful of any allergies!) You'd be surprised how many of us have old mismatched gloves lying around the house but gloves may be found for very little money at Salvation Army/Goodwill Stores, and for free in lost-and-found boxes in schools and other public places. You will also need assorted fabrics, needles and thread or fabric glue, yarn, buttons, sense of humor, fabric markers.

–

How To

Glove puppets are not a new concept in art therapy, but rarely are they used to explore issues related to growing a positive body image. Because the metaphor of the hand can be interpreted in so many ways as it relates to food, love, self-soothing, holding on and letting go, the possibilities for using this activity are limitless. Here are a few suggestions of themes to help you explore your personal and unique journey on the road to self-acceptance:

- When you reach for something to eat, what are some of the things you are reaching for that are not related to the food?
- What are some positive things about your body and/or your life that you would like to hold onto?
- What new experiences or feelings would you like to grab onto?
- Who or what positive influences do you want to keep nearby and easily accessible in your life?

1. Now, trace your hand on a piece of paper to plan out what you would like your g(love) puppet to look like. Will you use the entire glove to express one complete image or create a glove with each finger representing something different? There is no right or wrong choice!

2. Once you have designed your puppet, use the materials you gathered and recreate a three dimensional version of your sketch. Remember, this is for YOU, so if you want to use glue that's great, if you want to sew, that's fine too. You may choose to put things in the palm of the glove that you want to hold on to and decorate the outside with what makes it difficult for you to do that. You may opt to decorate each finger as a factor that contributes to your emotional eating and the palm of the glove may have a symbol of what you can do to fulfill your needs differently. If you can imagine this activity as creating your own personal "helping hand", you will end up with a tangible reminder that you can slip into (literally or figuratively). When challenges arise and you want to get back on the track of self-acceptance and a less conflicted relationship with food, this can be…wait for it… very…handy.

—

Why

Punch and Judy, *Sesame Street*, Glovey in *Yellow Submarine*, and the infamous Shari Lewis' Lambchop are just a few examples of how hand puppets have been used in delightful ways to convey all kinds of messages. Pledges often involve placing our hand over our heart to indicate our dedication to the pledge, and the expression, my "heart is in my hand" professes open and authentic love to another person. Unless we have lost the use of our hands as a result of a disability, we typically use them to soothe a loved one or to reach for food. Hands can be an important metaphor when used in conjunction with the expressive heARTs.

Notes

Proactivity # 2

Spread the Word

Materials

Paper, pencils, pens, markers, collage materials, glue sticks, scissors. Optional: Access to the Internet.

—

How To

1. Choose one aspect of eating disorders or body image that you would like to share with people via a social media tool (e.g., Twitter, Facebook, Tumblr, Digg, email, Blog, etc). You can also try designing a logo/symbol for Eating Disorder awareness and include one specific reason why it is important to increase our own and others' awareness of ED's or Body Image Dysmorphia.

2. Choose which social media tool or tools you are going to design the information for, taking into account word limits, graphics, privacy considerations, et cetera.

3. Using the art materials you have available, design a "post" about your personal experience with an eating disorder or information about eating disorders/body image to share with someone who may either have an e.d., work with clients, or have a family member for whom eating disorders are an issue. This can be anything from creating a full Facebook page, a Pinterest photo, or as simple as a Tweet. When your piece is finished, if you feel comfortable share it with at least one other person either via social media or in person. I am always happy to receive your work at **drdeah@drdeah.com**. See what insights or questions emerge. What do you feel the other person/people learned from your piece?

4. If appropriate, post the finished work on a Social Media Site during February's National Eating Disorders Awareness Week.

—

Why

February's Eating Disorders Awareness Week provides us the opportunity to learn more about our own eating disorder/body image issues and/or to educate others. Sometimes, when we work on something for someone else, we are less inhibited because we want to help. Have you ever had the experience where you would do something for someone else before doing anything for yourself? This generosity of spirit and altruism frequently opens up information that is applicable and meaningful in our own personal journey to body positivity and self-acceptance.

Notes

MARCH
Spring Ahead

Personal Perspectives

> *And the seasons they go round and round...*
>
> –JONI MITCHELL

As spring approaches, I find myself thinking about the cyclical nature of life. This isn't very deep or profound; the circular pattern of the seasons is a classic topic of contemplation with a long history in poetry and prose. Depending on my frame of mind, this repetition or redundancy can trigger feelings of despair or being stuck in patterns that just won't budge. On the other hand, considering that spring is supposed to be about new beginnings, it may spark a sense of urgency for spring cleaning and a fresh start. Either way, spring inevitably adds additional pressure to someone who is trying to be patient with incremental change.

> *...We're captive on a carousel of time...*

When I am at my best, I find great comfort in this predictable repetition. Seeing the plum tree in my back yard begin to blossom right on target every March fills me with a sense of safety that, at least in this part of the planet, all is right with the world. And when something is predictable, it provides us with the opportunity to be proactive and prepare for what is ahead.

> *...We can't return we can only look behind from where we came...*

Each season has its own idiosyncratic obstacles for those of us on a journey to cultivate a healthier, happier body image, and spring is no exception. The Mexican novelist Augustin Jose wrote this about time:

> *...Yesterday is gone. Tomorrow has not yet come. We have only today. Let us begin.*

It is important to remember that our history is not our fate; it is knowledge. Yes, it can be a good indicator of what our tendencies are and what we have typically been inclined to do. It is not, however, a fait accompli, and we can learn from our past.

The month of March – and sometimes April (depending on how the dates fall during the year) – provides us with a substantial crop of opportunities, disguised as holidays, to practice this body-positive approach to living. One of these is Passover.

Passover is one of many Jewish holidays celebrated with a ritual feast. This feast is filled with symbolic foods and a prescribed schedule for which foods to eat when. Depending upon how observant the participants are, there is a wide range of recipes for the ritual readings at a Passover Seder. Some read from ancient texts, others from more progressive versions. Some are tailored for passionate political discussion, others for children with short attention spans. Despite the diversity of the Seder itself, there are at least three specific commonalities adhered to by the most Liberal and Orthodox Jewish celebrants alike:

- There is no leavening used in any of the meals.
- There are at least four cups of wine.
- When it is time to eat, there are no restrictions on how much you can eat.

As a kid growing up, dieting and caloric restrictions were an everyday part of my life. I was surrounded by dieters. The youngest of three girls, my two older sisters always dieted, and both of my parents did as well. The diets never really seemed to work – none of us were thin. My mother often chortled, "Imagine how fat we would all be if we didn't diet!"

And, of course, I believed her and followed suit.

Many young girls that diet wind up becoming sneak eaters, and I was no different. Because we are forced to satisfy our hunger and cravings privately, we develop the notion that we are beasts (roar!) with insatiable appetites. Our appetite for food feels freakish, and our need to satiate this hunger is so strong that we must adopt furtive methods of feeding the monster. We feel weak in our inability to resist the urges to eat the "bad" food, and yet, the part of us that is demanding the food is a formidable foe of great strength and power. As a result, we are split and fractured around food.

The Problem in a Nutshell: Passover and other food-centric holidays present a double bind for people already struggling with feelings about how and what they eat, how and what they don't eat, how and what they would like to eat if they were allowed to eat, and how and what they wished they had eaten when they had the chance.

I KNOW YOU HAVE TO READ THAT SENTENCE AGAIN…BUT TRUST ME IT MAKES SENSE!

The Double Bind of Passover: A Two-Act Play

Act I: The week before the Seder, we obsessed over what to wear in order to prepare for the unsanctioned but equally predictable ritual of Passover…

The Body Scan: Everyone was always checking you out to see how you "measure up" to the last time you were all together. In my family, despite the fact that very few of us were thin, there was still a hierarchy within the ranks with clear labels. The "Always Thins" – they were the winners. Praise and attention were lavished on them like buttuh on the matzoh and our jealousy dripped like honey into a nice cup of tea.

Then there were the "Always Fats." They were already "fat's accompli." They would always be fat and that was that: "Those poor people."

The "Newly Thins" were the ones I envied the most. The attention they received, the fawning, the exclamations of "How did you do it? You look amazing!" They were the stars of the night. Somehow they had conquered the inner beast. They had become successful.

The "Fat Agains" were, conversely, the lowest caste of the crew. Also known as the "YO YOs," these were the mishpucha (family) who had lost but gained their weight back plus more. The "tsks tsks" and "cluck clucks" of the tongues, the subtle shakes of the heads, the implied message of "If I had lost that weight I would have kept it off," or more blatantly, "I knew s/he couldn't do it." They were the ones my heart ached for and the club I dreaded ever joining. (Of course I was in and out of that club numerous times, and sadly it wasn't until years later that I realized it was the dieting that actually created and perpetuated the problem.)

Act II: Off I would go to the Seder, "ready for my close up Mr. De Mille," dressed to the nines and encased like a blintz in belly-binding control-top panty hose. But the second bind of the double bind was not far away. After the reading of the ritual story of Passover, the feast would commence. Places everyone! But wait! It was as if they had replaced the cast with all new people and all new scripts.

All of a sudden, size and weight were inconsequential. There was a resounding chorus of, "Eat! Eat!" And, "Have more! What, you don't like my matzo balls? This is no time to diet, this is Passover, forget about it for just one night, you look fine!" and for the next couple of hours I felt normal. I felt happy. I felt I could eat with abandon and enjoyment. I could savor the pleasure of food, slowly, languidly and not worry whether I was leaving crumbs behind like a guilty Gretel who subconsciously wanted to get caught eating Ring Dings in her bedroom.

I didn't feel insatiable or monstrous. I didn't feel "wrong." I felt calm, and I felt in control. I had PERMISSION!

Why was this night different from all other nights?

Because on this night, I was, allowed to eat my fill in public. Now the double bind along with the control-top panty hose, are gone and replaced with self-acceptance and a healthier relationship with food every day.

And now, there is one less reason why this night IS different from all other nights!

Predictable Challenges

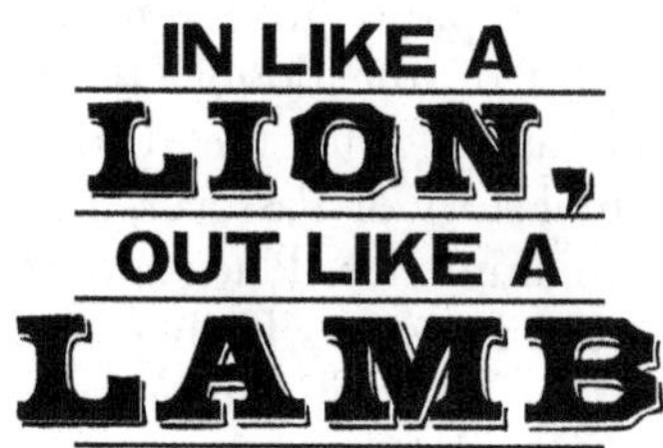
IN LIKE A
LION,
OUT LIKE A
LAMB

Such is the reputation of the month of March. Weather fluctuations aside, March is a month when the symbolism of dualities and transitioning is evident with formidable tests awaiting those of us with body dissatisfaction and or eating disorders.

As people begin shaking off their winter coats and emerging from their layers of down and sweaters, the prospect of more skin showing becomes a reality. This may trigger body-image panic to come out of hibernation and an overwhelming urge to "do something drastic" in the guise of spring cleaning. We can ameliorate some of these urges by taking a proactive approach. So let's look at some of the associations with spring:

- Spring is the season most associated with rebirth, reemerging from sleep, and perennials re-blooming.
- Springs of water replenish and circulate. Springs are not stagnant.
- When someone has a "spring in their step," it means they have bounce and positive energy.
- Spring coils have the power to propel.

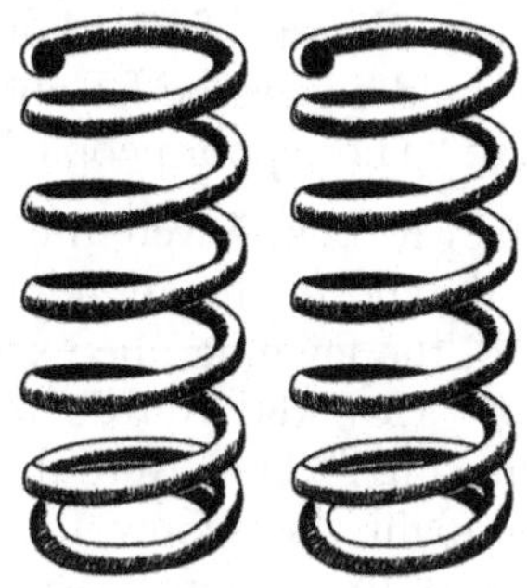

When we look at a spring, we see that, although it is circular and gives the impression of redundancy and repetition, it also has the sense of upward movement, support, and resiliency.

So, while we may be tempted to go from one extreme to another – from hibernation to full action – let's remember that this is a time of transition and thoughtful movement. No flower blooms overnight, even though that may seem to be the case. As we let go of old habits and behaviors that are self-destructive or reinforce our negative self-image and impair our self-acceptance, let's remember to hold on to the aspects of ourselves that are working in our favor. This is NOT an all-or-nothing proposition. Let's use our inner strength and self-devotion as foundations and spring boards to healthier relationships with food and a blossoming acceptance of the wonders of our body's natural shape.

Some things to consider:

- There may be a compulsion to start a restrictive diet with the onset of the warmer weather.
- Fear of bingeing related to St. Patrick's and other religious food-centric rituals may be anxiety provoking for those with eating disorders.
- Beware of an onslaught of ads by diet companies promoting programs promising quick and magical transformations. Messages like "Springing into the NEW YOU" are tailored to result in self-loathing with the only cure being extreme restrictive dieting or quick-fix weight loss surgery interventions.

Important Dates to Remember

- First week of March – Love Your Body Week at Chico State University, California
- March 8 – International Women's Day
- The entire month of March is Women's History Month.

All of these occasions invite us, men and women alike, to take some time to celebrate women's accomplishments over the years. Let's take time to identify aspects of ourselves worthy of honoring and appreciating.

- March 17 – St. Patrick's Day is touted as an alcohol- and food-laden celebration. The media, and frequently our peers, encourage binge drinking, which may impair mindful and intuitive eating.
- Spring equinox dates vary but fall between March 20-25, allowing us to tap into the possibilities of healthy ways to spring forward, and to revel in the beautiful diversity of sizes and shapes present in all of nature's forms. Blossoms, whether tiny and delicate or big and flamboyant, all have a place in the garden.
- Passover, Purim, and Easter dates vary but typically fall between the third week of March or later (sometimes into April). These are typically holidays with a strong emphasis on ritual feasts and traditional foods.

(And just as an aside, did you know that March is both National Nutrition Month AND National Frozen Food Month?!! Talk about duality!)

First week in March – Love Your Body Week (Chico State University, California
March 8th – International Women's Day
March 17th – St. Patrick's Day

Proactivity # 1

Spring Gleaning

Materials

Basic variety of art supplies for collage and/or drawing, including but not limited to: paper, pens, pencils, markers, magazines, scissors, glue sticks.

–

How to

1. Sit quietly for a few minutes and contemplate the expression, "In like a lion, out like a lamb." If that phrase was applied to you, what words would you use to describe how you entered winter and how you are emerging into spring?

2. Using collage and/or drawing media, create a representation of the "before" status on one side of the paper and the "after" image on the other side. You can also use two completely separate pieces of paper.

3. Now focus on the transition itself – the "middle ground," so to speak. Which parts of you will you hold onto as you spring into the new season? Which parts of you would you like to leave behind? Why?

4. Either on the same piece of paper or on a third piece of paper, create a representation of this "middle ground."

5. When the piece is complete, see if there are any tangible items that you would like to add to your body-positive "To Do" list – and if you are really motivated and have continued to create your monthly "Adventure Calendar" (see January) – write them down and add to the pouches on the days of the month.

–

Why

There is a fine line between self-evaluation and renewal and the compulsion for a TOTAL MAKEOVER. Unfortunately, our society promotes the latter, leading people with body dissatisfaction and eating disorders to cave into the media pressure to "SPRING into the NEW YOU," diet our old selves away, and strip away winter fat through surgery and starvation. But we have choices. When we emerge into spring, there are wonderful aspects of ourselves that we can opt to hold onto, cultivate, and nurture. This activity is designed to facilitate the exploration of the fertile middle ground that the transition into spring offers.

Notes

Proactivity # 2

Positive Posters

Materials

Poster board, sketch paper, magazines, markers, pencils, paint, glue sticks, scissors. Optional: personal photographs.

–

How To

1. Sit quietly for a moment and think about the fact that March is the "month of the woman" and has been designated to celebrate the accomplishments of women all over the world and throughout history.

2. Have a piece of paper and a pencil handy and imagine you are designing a poster that illustrates some of your accomplishments over your lifetime. Jot down the ones that come to mind.

3. Remember that the accomplishment does NOT have to be world changing or lifesaving! It can just be something that has had a positive effect on your or someone else's life. Select one or more events to include on your poster.

4. Sometimes, our self-esteem is so tenuous that it may be difficult to identify one single event. Don't stress over this. It's not unusual for those of us who have body dissatisfaction to feel unsuccessful in other areas in our lives. That is why we are here doing this work! If this is the case, make a poster for someone else who has impacted your life in a positive way.

5. With the materials provided, go to work. I mean, play! Create your posters. Remember, there is no "right" or "wrong" way to design your poster. If you want to do a practice design on scratch paper first, that's fine, too. Words, images, anything goes!

6. If you did a poster about someone else, see if you can identify the quality of that person that you found worthy of acknowledging and consider whether or not someone would look at you and feel that you also embodied that quality or trait. Could someone feel the same way about you?

–

Why

Taking time to acknowledge our strengths and the positive changes we have made in our own lives or someone else's, is often very difficult; yet, it is vital for growing a more positive body image, reevaluating our priorities, and introducing movement into our stagnant thought patterns. All too often, we are accustomed to using our weight, dress size, or calorie count as the one and only barometer for what makes us a successful person. We forget about the other aspects of who we are and how, at any size or any weight, we have a great deal to be proud of.

Notes

APRIL
Constant Comments

Personal Perspectives

I am not clear how this came about … but about … it certainly came.

There seems to be an unspoken rule that it is perfectly okay for people to comment on other people's bodies. And I am not referring only to the behind-the-back conspiratorial comments frequently accompanied by a wink wink nudge nudge to a nearby co-commenter. I am not even talking about the never-ending stream of body comments in the tabloids. I am talking about face-to-face, full-body-slam-contact commenting by strangers who feel perfectly justified in walking up to someone and letting them know that they are fat. A public service announcement of immense proportions doled out as if I had been living my life under a rock:

> *No, really??? Me??? Why, I hadn't noticed! Thanks for telling me that…now I will fix it and my whole life will be better, and all because of you!*

> *Oh wait! Don't leave! How in the world can I ever repay you?*

And then there are those who are more specific in their assault as they single out a particular body part that they find offensive or distasteful:

> *Wow, you'd be such a babe if you lost some of that fat around your middle.*

To which the thought that inevitably crosses my mind is:

> *I'm sorry … but have we met????*

And it's not even the incidents involving strangers that are the most egregious. What about the times when you are with someone and you feel safe, loved, and sexy? Someone with whom you have shared intimate moments with … sans clothes … who suddenly finds it vital to inquire whether or not you have considered losing some weight in order to be really beautiful? Did I miss the amendment to the etiquette constitution that afforded people the right to give their unsolicited opinion about my body?

Where are the filters between thought and speech that most of us were taught growing up? You know the ones:

- Think before you speak.
- If you don't have something nice to say, just don't say it.
- Do unto others as you would have them do unto you.

I can't remember ever going up to someone and saying:

> *Wow, you'd be great if you just dyed your hair a different color or grew six inches.*

(Apply that six-inch comment to any part of the body you'd like!)

On any given day, there is an avalanche of news stories about bullying. Most of the attention is typically focused on situations involving race, sexual orientation, or religion, and include tips for intervening. One explanation that experts offer is that most bullies were abused and are perpetuating the abuse cycle with their own bullying behaviors. The victims are offered support as well, and they are being counseled to speak up and not suffer in silence. Schools and workplaces are implementing zero-tolerance policies along with both proactive and consequential strategies to eliminate bullying cultures. And I applaud this trend wholeheartedly.

But what about the situations where the targets are peoples' body size? When the targets for the bullies are fat, there seems to be no attempt to enlighten the bully about the error of their ways, and the advice is almost certain to be directed at the victim and usually sounds something like:

> *Just lose the weight and then you won't be a target.*
>
> *You are just asking for it by not losing weight.*
>
> *The best revenge will be getting thin, that will show him!*

These attitudes are insidious in a variety of ways, but one of the most destructive is that it implies that there is nothing wrong with shaming a person for being fatter than the bully's definition of what is NOT too fat. With society's message internalized, many of the victims of fat bullying don't feel it is appropriate to stand up to the perpetrator; instead, a common inner monologue goes something like this:

> *Guilty as charged! I am fat and deserve to be admonished for my crime against society. I am an eyesore in your world and if I walk out in public it means I have checked the box indicating that I accept the terms of agreement for being abused by total strangers.*

And so I continue on my quest and ask the same two QUEST(ions) I have been asking for so many years and no one has been able to answer:

- Why do we hate people just because they are fat?
- Why do people feel entitled to verbally abuse people because they are fat?

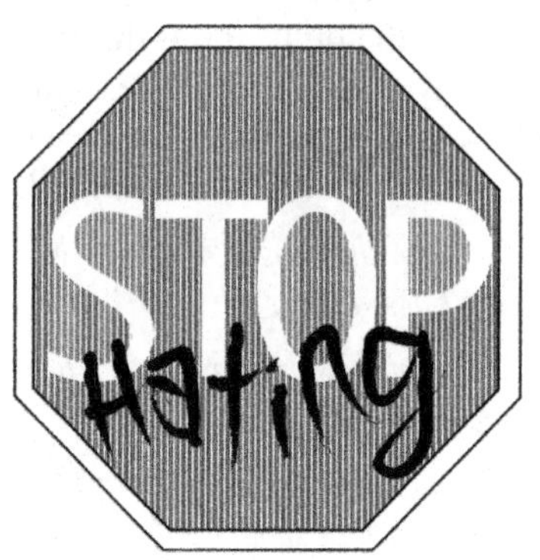

I am hungry for any public proclamation that calls for people to examine their prejudices and change their hateful points of view and actions. The same way that diversity training programs ask folks to examine their internalized racism, I would love it if people would acknowledge their bias against fat people and own up to their inner bully. Of course, in order to do that, we must believe that:

- People are capable of that level of insight.
- That insight leads to a change of behavior.

Those are assumptions that I find difficult to have faith in at times, but if I didn't believe in change of that magnitude, I would have thrown my therapist towel into the ring years ago. The gear shifting step from internal attitudinal change to external behavioral change is huuuuuuge, necessary and not easy. Once we admit that it is wrong to judge people based on their bodies and even "more wrong" to feel entitled to verbalize those opinions, we need to learn to speak up. I know, I know, that sounds contradictory – learn when not to speak and then learn to speak up – but think back and remember when we were learning what words we could and could not use in front of our grandmother, and trust that we still have that skill set!

Whether we are the victim, a reformed perpetrator, or the witness of fat bashing, it is our responsibility to cultivate our own constant comments that tell ourselves or others:

If you think you are helping, you are not.

Why are you being so mean?

Have you considered another point of view?

Funny, I don't recall asking for your opinion.

Changing another person's opinion or behavior is a daunting task. I am not suggesting that there will be immediate results by adopting an activist approach. But inaction rarely leads to change in others or ourselves.

As someone who admits freely to having my own share of control issues, I have had to accept that we may not be able to change someone else, but changing some aspects of ourselves is completely in our control. So while we continue to find ways to change the societal construct that allows people to body bash another person, we can, at the same time, examine our own self-bashing. We can begin to think twice before we initiate our self-hate inner monologue.

And you don't have to tackle this by yourself! There is an End Bullying Campaign that has been initiated by The National Association to Advance Fat Acceptance (NAAFA) in Southern California that is taking on size bullying and has a great curriculum available. For more information, contact naafa.org.

MY ONLY WEIGHT PROBLEM IS YOUR PROBLEM WITH MY WEIGHT

Predictable Challenges

April arrives on the scene with two predictable challenges for those of us cultivating our body positivity. The first is managing the full throttled media assault that comes as predictably as moving our clocks forward. It is in April that we are all supposed to start getting ready for bathing suit season. April, we are warned, means we have only two months to attain our bikini worthy bodies. With chocolate eggs and marshmallow Peeps still in abundance around us, the ads now chastise us for having indulged in our Cadbury Bunny Bites and are aggressively fertilizing our internal seeds of self-loathing. The media urges us to tune into the ominous beating of the distant drums of summer as they get louder and come closer. They fan the flames of our anxiety as the days of April pass by, and they are counting on us to believe that our one and only worthy goal is to lose the winter weight we all must have assuredly gained while hibernating in our caves. The objective is to convince us that we do not deserve to have fun unless our bodies are slimmer by summer and the only way to attain a bathing-suit-worthy body is by buying whatever it is they are trying to sell.

The second challenge that arises in April for some folks struggling with eating disorders and body dissatisfaction is spring break. Spring break often means less structure regarding work, school, and leisure activities. The welcomed extra free time may not always feel so welcome when it results in a resurgence of unconscious eating for those who tend to eat when they are bored or lonely. The pressure on college students to overindulge in alcohol, food, with reckless abandon – as dictated by the flood of movies that appear every year at this time – is enormous. This, in turn, may spur some feelings of being out of control. Self-destructive behaviors may be triggered in an attempt to manage those feelings and regain a sense of one's balance.

For families who rely on school meals as primary nourishment for their children, being at home may bring about a scarcity of food or a more limited choice of healthy food options.

"April is the cruelest month," wrote the poet T. S. Eliot in his poem *The Wasteland.* But the poem proceeds to describe April as a month where beauty and life spring from hardship, "breeding lilacs out of the dead land. Mixing memory and desire. Stirring dull roots with spring rain."

Using the approach of finding the positive side to potentially negative situations and nurturing our growing love for our bodies, will help us successfully navigate through the challenges of April. Remember that, despite the external media pressures, it is important to focus on what is happening inside.

- Check in with your feelings that arise with unstructured free time or peer pressure to over consume.
- Reinforce the importance of internal qualities and the beauty of body diversity.
- De-emphasize the importance of the scale and the mirror.
- Remember that diets do not work and mindful eating is a year-round practice.
- Explore enjoyable opportunities for physical activity for fun, not for weight loss, and to improve a sense of body competency.
- Use your support network to resist the temptation to buy into the negative messages and replace them with ones that are self-affirming and joyful. These interventions may not help you with your taxes (arguably the cruelest part of April for some), but they certainly will help proactively avoid a relapse or intensification of disordered eating and self-hate.

Important Dates to Remember

April is National Poetry Month, and for those who think that poets do not have a sense of humor, do you think it was an accident that members of the National Poet's Society have been known to distribute free copies of Eliot's *The Wasteland* to post offices around the country on Tax Day ... smack dab in the middle of April??

- April is also National Humor Month and National Stress Awareness Month
- April 1 – April Fool's Day
- April 30 – National Honesty Day (something about the symmetry of that amuses me)
- April 22 – Earth Day
- The dates of spring break vary, but

you can find more about managing the potential negative repercussions of Spring Break at the American College Health Association website: acha.org

April 1st – April Fool's Day
April 22nd – Earth Day
April 30th – National Honesty Day

Proactivity # 1

Pillow Talk

Materials

Plain white pillowcases, fabric paints and or fabric markers, (make certain you use fabric paints/markers that won't bleed when washed), scratch paper, and pencils.

–

How To

1. On scratch paper, draw at least one image of a positive internal quality that you are proud of or that makes you feel good about yourself.

2. Somewhere in the image, in honor of National Poetry Month, create a poem using the words, "It's what's on the inside that counts," or just use the words themselves.

3. Turn the pillowcase inside out.

4. Using fabric paints or markers, replicate the image from the scratch paper onto the pillowcase. (Remember the design and words are on the inside of the pillowcase. The outside of the pillowcase will remain undecorated.)

–

Why

To reinforce the concept that focusing on who we are on the inside carries more "weight" than our external appearance and conforming to societal standards of beauty.

Notes

Notes

Proactivity # 2

Self-Adooration

Materials

Manila file folder, collage materials, scratch paper, pens, paper, markers, scissors, glue sticks.

–

How To

1. Take a moment to sit quietly and imagine that the file folder, when looked at vertically, is a door that opens up. Behind the door is at least one thing that will help you stay centered during the month of April (when the pressures from the outside to get bathing-suit ready or anxieties related to spring break are mounting).

2. Using the art materials available, decorate the front of the file folder with some symbols of the pressures that you anticipate will be "banging at your door" during the month of April.

3. Open the folder, and decorate the inside depicting the strengths, support, plan, or strategy you can utilize to stay focused on maintaining your positive body self-esteem and/or healthy relationship with food.

–

Why

Using a door as a metaphor literally opens up doors to exploration of feelings and ways to manage those feelings. Doors also symbolize ways to keep out negative influences and welcome in positive ones. April is a month of increased negative media influence regarding body image and peer pressure to over consume alcohol and food during spring break. By predicting what the pressures will be and proactively preparing to manage them, we can choose not to succumb to old self-destructive patterns.

Notes

Notes

MAY
Momeries

Personal Perspectives

My mom hated her body. I knew this at a very young age, but I didn't understand it.

I loved my mom's body – not just for all of the reasons that so many of us write about: the enveloping arms and squishy soft pillows of comfort offered for snuggles and consoling. I also loved my mom's body because I saw it as constant, immortal, forever there, and always accessible. Her size and shape had nothing to do with my love for her body. My love was about attachment. My love was about unconditional availability. My love was without eyes or judgment.

So when I heard my mom complaining about her butt and thighs, I was bothered.

When I heard my mom crying in the bathroom and I'd peek in and see her crying in front of the mirror, I was bewildered.

When I saw her taking the combination of blue and red capsules out of the little white boxes that Dr. Wortman used to give her, I was be…

(Ooh, this is starting to sound like a Rodgers and Hart song … *Bewitched, Bothered and Bewildered* was I!)

Actually, I was scared. I didn't understand the pills, the tears, or the hatred she clearly had for herself.

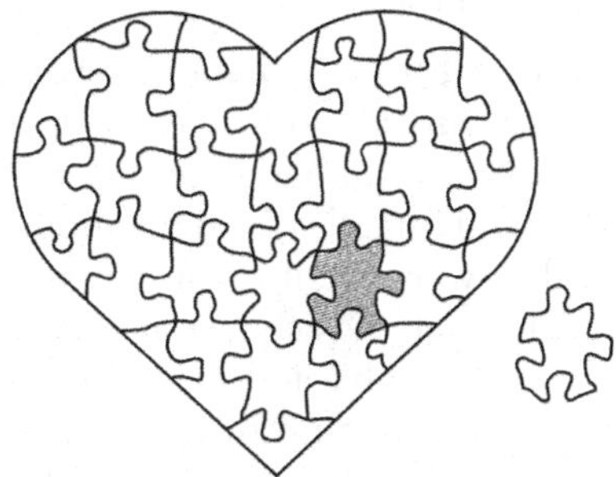

It was incongruent with my experience of loving her so much – like a puzzle missing a piece.

My mother wore army boots. Literally … she wore army boots. She wore overalls, army boots, and she was years before her time. She sent my sister and me to school with backpacks way before they were popular. We hated her for it. We wanted pretty little book bags. We got army surplus backpacks. Later on, in the late 1960s, we were the coolest with our symbolic anti-war army jackets and rucksacks, but by then, it was too late. It is hard to feel cool when we had lived so many years feeling just a tad ashamed of Mom's eccentricities.

When I was 13, my mom died of leukemia. She got sick in October, 1969, and died two months later. By then, I had adopted her body hate as my own. I had incorporated her habits of crying over the bathroom scale, wearing big cover-up clothing, and being embarrassed about my body. I, too, was taking pills. No Dr. Wortman for me. These were illegally obtained from some high school kid. They were white and had little crosses on them.

By the age of 15, I had grown to hate my Mom's body because it became my body. I had inherited some wonderful qualities from my mother, but they were totally eclipsed by the negative genetic legacy she passed on to me. I inherited her shortness, her roundness, and sturdiness. I had not been given any examples of how to love my body. I grew up brainwashed by the message that this was a body to despise: In other words, I was TAUGHT to hate my body.

Years later, I would realize that what I really hated was how abandoned I felt when she died. The betrayal, and the reality that this wonderful, precious, irreplaceable, Mommy Body was gone forever ... it was easier to hate my thighs than to really grieve the loss.

Our bodies are so much more than circumference and pounds. They are literally vessels for our spirit, allowing us to hold, hug, support, and love each other in <u>this</u> realm. I am not sure what happens to us after we die, but one thing I know for certain: face to face, eye to eye, hug to hug contact disappears with that person when someone dies.

Ma died when she was 52. When I turned 52, I opened up my Mom-ory Box. It was filled with my mom's trinkets, cards, and clothing. In the box were the overalls that she used to wear. They had embroidered flowers on the bib, and white lace stitched onto the legs. They were kind of girly girl, in a way. They were, I realized for the first time, a size 14. My mom suffered a life time of self-loathing as a size 14. I put them on. They fit just right.

I looked in the mirror and grinned. I looked adorable! Like a 52-year-old Pippi Longstocking! I stood there and cry-iled – you know, that crying and smiling at the same time thing we do when both emotions are equally powerful and you have to call it a tie?

I closed my eyes and decided to give myself permission to love my mom's and my body, for the two of us, as fervently as I could. I wore those overalls most of the day until I went out for my birthday dinner.

(My mom would have worn them into Chez Panisse, or French Laundry, but I wasn't that brave!) Still I carried my mom to dinner with me that night, in my thighs, my butt, my belly, and my heart.

I remember the first Mother's Day without my child at home. He was a college freshman 3,000 miles away, yet he dutifully "CAWLED HIS MUTHUH." Our conversation meandered effortlessly from topic to topic, giggles, tears, politics, and school. We are very close, very chatty, and unashamed to acknowledge how much we love each other.

I inherited that quality from my mom. My son knows that I am constant, forever there, and always accessible. My size and shape have nothing to do with our relationship. He loves me without eyes or judgment. And equally as important, I feel the same way about myself.

May is a very complicated month. It starts off with International No Diet Day on May 6th and ends with Memorial Day on the last Monday. Smack dab in the middle is Mother's Day. Let's take them one at a time.

Predictable Challenges

INTERNATIONAL NO DIET DAY. On May 6, one week before Mother's Day, there's a lesser-known holiday to mark on your calendar. Founded in 1992 by Mary Evans Young, director of Britain's Diet Breakers, International No Diet Day (INDD) is an annual tribute to body acceptance and body shape diversity. This day is also dedicated to promoting a healthy lifestyle and raising awareness of the dangers and futility of repeat dieting (a.k.a. weight cycling).

The goals of INDD:

- Question the belief that there is only one "right" body shape.
- Raise public awareness of weight discrimination, size bias, and fatphobia.
- Educate others by providing facts about the diet industry and emphasize the failure of commercial diets.
- Show how diets perpetuate violence against women.
- Honor the victims of eating disorders.
- Declare a day free from restrictive weight loss diets and obsessions with body weight, and try these thoughts on for size:

TODAY... I will love my body without apologizing or justifying.

TODAY... I will be more than a number on a scale.

TODAY... I will enjoy what I am eating without beating myself up.

TODAY... I will love my thighs for all that they are and not apologize for what they are not.

TODAY... I will move for the sheer pleasure of moving and will not check to see how many calories I burned.

TODAY... I will not spend precious time away from my friends and family calculating weight/calorie ratios or purging what I just ate.

TODAY... I will mind less about my size and mind more about my mind.

TODAY... I will rest my brain from the judgments, comparisons, and promises about what my body should look like.

In retrospect, I remember how exhausting it was to just carry the weight of my obsession around with me every minute of every day, never believing it was possible to let go of my concerns for just ONE DAY. Not just the food obsession – the thin obsession as well.

Restrictive dieting is designed to be failure oriented, and it shifts our attention away from pleasurable, mindful eating, joyful movement, and acceptance of who we are now. When we are being served the same messages day in and day out, it is easy to forget that we are allowed to order something different off the menu. The diet mentality and its associated self-hatred is a difficult habit to break.

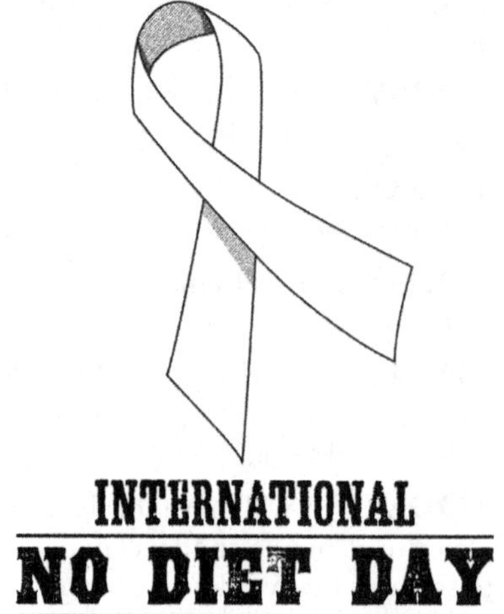

Difficult, but not impossible.

So relax ... It's just ONE DAY. Enjoy it!

MOTHER'S DAY. Perhaps it is a coincidence, and perhaps it is because I called my mother "Ma," but the first two letters of "May" remind me that MAy brings us Mother's Day. Despite the fact that some folks tout this as a shamelessly commercial "Hallmark" opportunity for selling cards and gifts, others experience it as a more poignant day, rife with meaning and fertile ground for insight and growth.

In the realm of food and body image, the connections between mothering, nourishment, nurturing, and the female body are easily accessible during this time. You don't have to be Freud or even Freudian to understand that looking at our earliest associations with food, love, and self-soothing MAY provide us with valuable information about our current relationship with food and our bodies in the present. Our mothers are frequently the first mirror we have about the importance and meaning of food and our bodies. Powerful role models, we choose to either emulate our mothers or rebel against them, consciously or unconsciously. How we integrate the messages we received from our moms impacts our behaviors and self-image long after we have left the nest.

Whether or not we have any kids of our own, we are all still mothers to ourselves each and every day. As adults, we have the honor and awesome responsibility of taking care of ourselves and must learn how to discern between the positive mothering skills we learned from our mothers and those less beneficial to our physical and emotional health. This MAY be an opportunity to do some spring cleaning and discard some less healthful behaviors, beliefs, or habits, while showing gratitude for the ones that are enriching our lives. Once again, I need to point out that this isn't always easy to do – especially if we're prone to guilt.

How can I reject my mother???

If I do it differently than my mother, what does that say about how I feel about my mother?

I would like to take three giant steps please! Ack! I didn't say, "Mother, may I?" I have to go back to the starting line!

(For those of you too young to remember, "Mother, May I?" is a game similar to "Simon Says." You had to ask permission to move forward. And if you got almost all the way to the finish line and forgot to ask, "Mother may I?" you had to go all the way back to the starting line. No room for error. All or nothing.)

At a certain point in our lives, however, we are allowed to move forward without obtaining permission from our mother and we can choose from a variety of mothering styles, ranging from overly detached ("othering") to overly enmeshed ("smothering"). Consciously choosing a different style than our mothers used is not necessarily disrespectful, nor does it diminish the loving intentions that hopefully accompanied their actions. We MAY choose to let go of some aspects of how we were mothered and keep others.

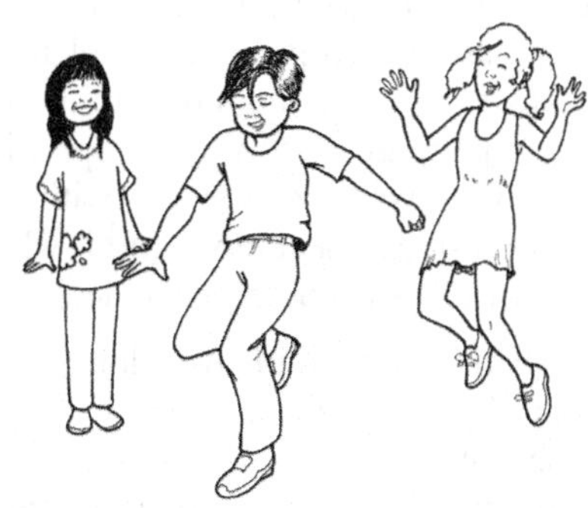

I will resist all temptation to make a pun about being my mother's keeper and instead propose that it is never too late to learn how to be a good mom to ourselves and take good care of our bodies, minds, and spirits. This means learning how to provide a supportive, nurturing, and accepting environment for growth and sustenance. A stretch? Yes! Complex? You bet! Look at what we are up against!

EMOTIONAL EATING IS ALWAYS A NO NO!

One of the negative outcomes of our diet-obsessed culture is what a bad rap "emotional eating" has gotten from the dieting industry. Under the auspices of health and good parenting, we have deified food restriction. We are told that if we EVER eat when we are NOT hungry or to self-soothe or celebrate, that somehow we have failed in our quest to achieve that coveted prize: a detached and apathetic relationship with food. But we are human. And, from the very start, our experiences with food are intertwined with love and emotions; sad and joyous occasions. To place a completely negative value judgment on eating for emotional reasons is in direct opposition to what we have grown up with. It is a confusing expectation, and is why so many of us become yo-yo dieters.

I wish my mom had lived longer. I think I could have helped her; because unlike my mom, I became bilingual in the languages of food and love. I adopted a more mindful relationship with eating that helps me understand the difference between hunger, appetite, and satiety and doesn't exclude any one category out of fear.

I slowly re-taught myself that self-acceptance, health, and self-worth are NOT based on being thin enough or weighing a certain amount. I no longer use my body as a way to garner acceptance and approval from others.

Am I saying it's been a cake walk? Absolutely not! I have had to learn how to trust myself with food instead of adopting punitive, restrictive diet plans and extreme doctrines that call for an all-or-nothing approach. These interventions inevitably set us up for bingeing and self-loathing. Our bodies and brains become the arena for the war between the "loving moms" who give us permission to eat more than our fill, and the nagging, punitive mom hollering,

> *YOU DIDN'T SAY "MOTHER MAY I!!!!"*

I am not sure what my son, would say about my mothering skills. He doesn't read my blog. (I will guilt trip him about that later.) But I try my best to be a good mom to him and to me, and that means putting my beliefs of what makes a good mom into action. And, when I mess up I continue from where I am. I do not go back to the starting line. I believe that a good mom:

- Accepts their child for who they are. They reinforce their strengths, teach them how to be safe, and try to reshape and dissuade them from self-destructive or hurtful habits and behaviors.
- Teaches and role models tolerance and acceptance of diversity in others, and themselves.
- Realizes that a child must be nurtured, nourished, loved, and taught how to love and nourish themselves in the absence of the mom.
- Realizes that there is a middle ground – that no one is all good or all bad. And if you make a mistake, you don't have to go all the way back to the starting line.

Important Dates to Remember

Memorial Day is the last Monday in May and officially heralds the coming of summer. The weekend is often filled with picnics and mixed messages of feasts and celebrations as long as you are bathing-suit-ready for June … which is about a week away. This can cause a great deal of anxiety and may trigger a resurgence of binge eating or restrictive eating in order to cope.

It is helpful to think of Memorial Day as a time to remember: Remember to focus on your personal definition of self-acceptance. Stay mindful that the messages being directed at you are designed to lower your self-worth and that you can hold your course and stay in concert with your body. Remember that every day is a new opportunity to revel in who you are in this moment and NOT who you could be at some weight in the future.

Other important dates in May to consider:

- May 6 – INDD: healthateverysize-blog.org/2012/05/06/the-haes-files_international-no-diet-day
- May 9 – Children's Mental Health Awareness Day: nctsn.org
- National Mental Health Month: nmha.org
- May 12-18 – National Women's Health Week: womenshealth.gov
- Second Sunday in May – Mother's Day

May 6th – International No Diet Day
May 9th – Children's Mental Health Awareness Day
Second Sunday – Mother's Day

Proactivity # 1

My Mother, Myself

Materials

Large pieces of drawing paper, magazines, markers, colored pencils, scissors, glue sticks, lined writing paper.

—

How To

1. Using the lined writing paper, take a moment and brainstorm about ways you already physically, emotionally, and spiritually mother yourself.

2. Identify which of these are working and which may be having a less beneficial effect.

3. Using a tree or a garden as a metaphor (it is spring, after all) create a drawing or collage that depicts yourself flourishing from the positive mothering you are providing for yourself, and "weed" out the habits that are no longer helping you to thrive. Be specific. (Feel free to use any other metaphor if the garden or tree image doesn't resonate with you.)

4. Now, looking at the less helpful habits or mothering actions you use, problem-solve ways to weed those out and identify some potential replacements.

5. Remember that there are all different types of mothering styles, and choosing a different way than your mother used while you were growing up does not necessarily diminish your mom's loving intentions.

—

Why

Whether or not we have any of our own children, we are mothers to ourselves. Sometimes, how we take care of ourselves may have made perfect sense when we first started these behaviors, but now they are less beneficial, and can be left behind. This activity provides us with sacred time to explore the ways we already take good care of ourselves. What positive mothering skills have we incorporated from our mothers, and which ones no longer serve our physical and emotional health? What are some alternative self-care, self-affirming habits to adopt that are appropriate in the present? This is an opportunity to do some spring cleaning of our outdated habits and show gratitude for the ones that are enriching our lives.

Notes

Proactivity # 2

Peace TrEATy

Materials

A copy of the International No Diet Day (INDD) Pledge, (see below), drawing paper, markers, pencils, crayons, collage materials, Optional: Calligraphy pens (materials can be as simple or as expansive as you would like).

–

How To

1. Read the pledge for International No Diet Day (see below).

2. Choose at least one of the components that you feel you want to commit to for just one day. Or make up your own.

3. Create a treaty, complete with seal, signature, and witness signing. Heck – use a feathered pen and calligraphy to make the treaty if you want to. Have fun with it! Make it official!

4. At the end of the day, either draw, write, or make a collage about how it felt throughout the day to be abiding with your INDD treaty. What were the high points? What were the low points? What was easy? What was difficult? Most importantly, what were the reasons behind the barriers that may have come up for you that made it difficult?

5. Decide if there is a component about the INDD pledge that you would like to try the next day. Is it the same one or a different one? If not, why? If yes, leave your art and/or writing materials available to make a new treaty in the morning.

Special Note: There is no correct or incorrect outcome to this directive. This is about learning more about your personal barriers, speed bumps, red and green lights that affect your personal peaceful relationship with your body and/or relationship with food.

–

Why

When we call a truce for just one day in our war with our bodies and food, it gives us the opportunity to see what other options are available. What do our minds and bodies do when we are not primarily focused on what we look like, what we want to look like, who looks better than us, what we are allowed to eat, what is forbidden? This is a one-day declaration of peace with no pressure; a day to examine and explore an alternative paradigm.

INDD Pledge:

- I will attempt to not diet for one day, on May 6, International No Diet Day.
- Instead of trying to change my body to fit someone else's standards, I will accept myself just as I am.
- I will feed myself if I'm hungry.
- I will feel no shame or guilt about my size or about eating.
- I will think about whether dieting has improved my health and well-being or not.
- I will try to do at least one thing I have been putting off "until I lose weight."

Notes

JUNE
For Dads

Personal Perspectives

Daddy, am I pretty?

For many daughters, their fathers are the reflection of how a girl is perceived physically. For the dad, it's a powerful position to be in and not always the easiest to navigate. Because we live in a world where media pressure continues to measure success with a tape measure and a scale, knowing whether or not to compliment or comment on their daughter's appearance can cause a great deal of confusion. I have armloads of empathy for fathers who may feel lost in the Paternal Cul De Sac from Hell, trying to find their way out:

How can I help my daughter feel good about herself if I don't tell her she is pretty?

It's true that the world we live in makes it difficult; but imagine what kinds of things a dad would tell his son to help him feel good about himself that have nothing to do with being pretty or handsome. But sometimes, we hear:

But no one will like her if she's fat. I'm just looking out for her own good.

Would you want her to be in a relationship with someone who is that superficial? Is being in a relationship with someone else more important than having a healthy relationship with herself?

Okay, forget about that. How can I help my daughter love herself if I don't tell her to lose weight? After all, if her father doesn't tell her, who will?

That's an easy one…EVERYBODY!

Okay, I'll tell my daughter she is beautiful no matter what she weighs or looks like.

This shows indisputable good intentions but this too can be a mistake.

HUGE sigh of exasperation.

I know it seems unfair, but comments such as these still put the emphasis on her body and appearance and qualifies her self-worth through the arena of beauty.

I can't do anything right in this arena, can I?

Let's turn that around and ask the question a different way.

What can I do that is right in this arena?

So glad you asked! Can we stop using the word arena now???

Number 1: Recognize your power ...use it wisely.

(Wow, I sound like YODA!) Power you have...use it wisely you should.

Please understand how much influence you have as a father and take this aspect of parenting VERY seriously. I am not saying that there are no father-son issues that are also potentially problematic, but that there are father-daughter-specific pitfalls that arise when it comes to a girl's body image, and the stakes are high.

Case in point: I was 13 when my mother died, and my father was left alone to raise his daughters. Girls are super impressionable in their early adolescence, and 13 is a crucial age for developing a healthy body image. I was no different. I was already self-conscious about the transformation that was taking place ... my body seemed to be betraying me in so many ways. I could no longer be "one of the boys" in my t-shirts and jeans, climbing trees and playing ball – I had these breasts to contend with. I could no longer be invisible. My body became a place where uninvited comments crashed my private party of self-worth and comfort. My dad's concerns about my (actually completely normal developmental) weight gain during puberty complicated the issue. Then I started dieting and gained even more weight.

And so it began. I was praised when I was thin and shamed and pitied when I was fat. I didn't have a stable internal compass of who I was. There was no (self-esteem) needle always pointing north; it changed at any given time based on my body size and fluctuating weight. My father's opinions about my attractiveness carried even more – dare I say weight – when I started to be interested in boys. So, in order to please my dad, and all other males by proxy, I had to look a certain way, even though there was no way I could pull it off without dieting and diet pills.

Being healthy wasn't enough. I needed to be thin or I was a failure.

Of course, my dad was certain that his insistence was only more proof of his love for me, and I understand why he would feel that way. But as an adult, and a parent myself, I know now that the way he expressed his love for me and the manner in which I tried to earn his love – through my waistline – robbed me of any love I may have had for myself.

Number 2: Separation/Individuation

Becoming a parent was my first experience with the Occupy movement. It started with Occupy Womb, and spread like wildfire to Occupy Bedroom, Occupy House, Occupy Mind, and continues in the present to occupy my heart and my life. Never before had I felt so completely responsible for another person's happiness. Never before had another person's happiness been so integral to my own happiness. I wanted desperately to provide an environment where value and self-worth were not measured by waist size or pounds on the scale. I wanted to sever the cord that attached physical appearance to self-love and self-acceptance. But, even if we could raise our children in a completely weight-neutral attitudinal vacuum, one day, our kids will leave home or turn on the TV and, inevitably, they will be at a loss as to how to deal with the onslaught of this crazy, sexist, body-obsessed world.

Thus, the weight-neutral vacuum intervention (WNVI) is really not the way to go. Instead, it is important to offer counter messages and opposing views, and to cultivate an inquisitive mind that will question the norms. Two of these norms are (1) the belief that diets work and (2) that what you look like is more important than what kind of person you are. It is imperative to remember that your daughter's body is NOT your body; so please resist the impulse to put her on a diet and try with all of your might not to associate your love for her with her appearance.

Number 3: Fire the Judge

There is a difference between judging and exercising good judgment. As parents, we want to help our children learn to use good judgment as they figure out their lives. Poor body image and eating disorders go hand in hand. Think about this: If self-worth wasn't constantly associated with beauty, do you think that body dysmorphic disorder would even exist? It all starts with judgment – or should I say, poor judgment – when girls are taught that beauty is their most valuable asset. It is easy for fathers to fall into the role of judge in a misguided attempt to help their daughters. For some, not doing this is difficult and may feel cognitively dissonant. But there will be enough people out there who are more than happy to take on the roles of judge, jury, and executioner, with your daughter's body playing the role of the accused. So, perhaps what she needs is supportive counsel, helping her define her life and self-worth using a different set of standards. I think you'd be perfect for the part!

These are not pretty concerns … whoops! (Classic Freudian slip: I meant to write "petty" and it came out "pretty"! Way to go, subconscious!) These are not petty or pretty concerns. They come from a place of wanting to be a good dad and wanting happiness and success for your daughter. But it takes conscious and careful execution of these intentions to produce a result that is congruent with your desires. So, with Father's Day coming up, along with all of the ties, coffee mugs, and ridiculous TV-remote-control-joke Father's Day cards, take a moment to appreciate your daughter for being your daughter and enjoy a moment of precious, unconditional, and mutual love. It is a gift that will last forever.

Predictable Challenges

June is a month of transitions. School is out for summer and many families are partaking in promotions and graduations. Some folks are switching from a regulated schedule to a more chaotic one. Perhaps parents are adjusting to their college kids being back in the home or their younger children going away to camp or other summer programs. With new jobs for some and more free time for others, few people enter summer without experiencing some kind of shift from their normal routine. Transitions are difficult for many struggling with eating disorders and body image issues.

The stress generated from June's transitions often result in an increase of disordered eating and body dissatisfaction. So, let's dust off our "crystal ball" and predict the challenges that summer may bring, so we can plan ways to manage the stress and anxiety that change introduces into our lives.

Hello Mudder, Hello Fodder

The third Sunday in June is Father's Day. I know we just made it through Mother's Day and explored the symbolism and associations with mothering. Father's Day, for most, may not be as symbolically intense and loaded with emotional meaning as Mother's Day. The archetype of the Mother is perhaps more far reaching than that of the Father, but that doesn't mean that we are without fodder for growth, especially in light of the role a dad can play in his daughter's self-image, as we just discussed.

Boys are not completely spared from these early body image messages, especially if they are not developing stereotypically athletic bodies. Fathers may be less diplomatic with their sons than their daughters in dishing out negative body talk, figuring their son should "man up," take the criticism, and just do something about it. But did you know that the number of boys and men with body dissatisfaction and eating disorders has been steadily increasing over the past decade? So, boys and girls alike have their body image and self-perception shaped by messages from their fathers.

June also officially brings us the first day of summer. We have been working arduously since spring to reject the incessant barrage of media messages that "bathing suit season is coming!" Working on body positivity and size acceptance includes fostering the radical opinion that bathing suits exist primarily to allow us the option to swim in public facilities and everyone has a right to swim where they want to.

Wow! A revolutionary thought, no? Think about it. If a bathing suit is technically nothing more than the approved uniform for pools, lakes, and beaches, then everyone should be entitled to wear a suit and not be judged worthy or unworthy of baring their skin. But the hijacking of bathing suits by the fashion industry, and the sexist spin artfully orchestrated by magazines such as *Sports Illustrated*, has resulted in the cultural paradigm that "only people who look a specific way are allowed to wear a bathing suit in public." Isn't it maddening that the very same people who insist that fat people get off their "lard-asses" and get some exercise, in the same breath, make it taboo and shameful for them to do just that?

The meta message is that only thin people are allowed to swim in public. And while it isn't outright illegal for a fat person to wear a bathing suit at the local beach or pool, the shaming and bullying that inevitably is hurled at a fat person in a bathing suit has the same outcome: a fat-free environment. This level of discrimination is incredibly hurtful, to say the least, and managing our feelings of rejection and self-loathing is challenging. It is imperative that we remember that we have as much of a right as anyone else to feel good about our bodies. If we want to swim, surf, scuba dive, or sunbathe, it is our choice. No one should be allowed to take that from us.

And please, once again, don't forget that you are not alone. Working on improving our internal self-esteem and accepting our body is vital, but our body positivity grows stronger when coupled with a support system that reinforces this point of view.

Important Dates to Remember

Juneteenth, also known as Emancipation or Freedom Day, commemorates the announcement of the abolition of slavery in the US. This day symbolizes the power of civil rights movements and reinforces the importance of activism by all on behalf of those still oppressed. As long as any faction of our society is marginalized, we are all subject to being marginalized.

Third Sunday – Father's Day
June 19th – Juneteenth (Emancipation Day)

Proactivity # 1

Crystal Ball

Materials

Drawing paper, markers, and pencils.

–

How To

1. Take a moment, sit quietly, and think of one to three changes that you know will occur over the next three months.

2. Draw a large circle on your paper. This will be your "crystal ball." You will be using your crystal ball to look into the future for the next three months.

3. Using your art supplies, draw at least one but no more than three changes in your routine that will occur over the summer, and identify the feelings you predict will be generated from those changes.

When the drawing is complete, on a separate piece of paper write down the ways you imagine you will manage the feelings. Which ones are habitual? Which ones are counterproductive? What are some alternative ways to manage the feelings of stress and anxiety that accompany these changes in routine? If you are having difficulty identifying new coping strategies, don't be afraid to ask for help or see how other people are adjusting without using food or negative body thoughts as stress-management techniques.

–

Why

Frequently, one of the underlying issues of body dissatisfaction and disordered eating has to do with control. Transitions can be a trigger for feeling out of control. The stress that results needs to be managed. Predicting the challenges and identifying constructive coping strategies helps to regain a sense of control over the situation. When we plan options that are body positive, habitual negative body thoughts and restrictive dieting can be avoided. To recap, when we remove our body dissatisfaction and how we eat as the causes and the cures for feeling out of control, we can look directly at what is making us uncomfortable about this time of transition and more easily figure out how to regain our equilibrium.

Notes

Notes

Proactivity # 2

Freedom Flag

Materials

Paper, markers, pencils, glue sticks, scissors, or fabric and fabric paints, needle, thread.

–

How To

1. Take a moment, sit quietly, and think about some images that symbolize your independence from the "body police." What colors, shapes and or objects represent your body positivity and declare your equality? If you are more comfortable using words instead of graphic symbols, that is fine too.

2. Using a piece of scratch paper, design your flag.

3. Once you are satisfied with your design, replicate it either on paper or by using fabric. Remember, the flag can be any size you want.

–

Why

Flags carry a great deal of symbolism. If you explore the meaning behind a country, state, or organization's flag, you will see that nothing is chosen randomly: The colors, shapes, and figures used on the flag are rife with meaning. In creating a personal freedom flag, you are defining and proclaiming your freedom from the societal message that you have fewer rights than someone who has a more "acceptable" body. You are declaring your freedom and reinforcing your positive body identity.

Notes

Notes

JULY
Losing Wait

Personal Perspectives

Most of us have heard it. Many of us have said it. And sadly, the majority of Americans are still doing it.

"It" is waiting. Waiting to live our lives until our scale hits the magic number. Waiting to live our lives until we finally wriggle into the coveted dress size or effortlessly slip into (or out of) the "perfect" pair of jeans.

As a member of the baby boomer generation, I have become acutely aware of my aging process. This has been a slow revelation because there seems to be a glitch in the time-space continuum. I can't explain it, but I know it's there. For some inexplicable reason (where is Carl Sagan when you need him?), the generation ahead of me and the one behind me are all getting older. In my son's case, like some real life version of Joni Mitchell's song *Circle Game*, the years have indeed flown by and now MY boy is 20+. My dad is firmly planted in his 80s, and I haven't aged a day since college. Unfortunately, my body doesn't always agree with my perception of reality, and it has ways of telling me that I am not getting or staying any younger, and that time, indeed, waits for no one. Well, if time isn't waiting for me, then I am no longer willing to squander this opportunity to live my life fully and without apology.

Clearly, I need to lose some wait.

I know I am not writing about anything ground breaking or especially profound, but I feel compelled to remind people that it is time to take your wait problem seriously.

Why now?

Frequently, we establish these waiting patterns early in our lives when we are more impressionable to others' feedback and more invested in pleasing those around us. If we get the message that we don't look good enough or are too fat to swim, dance, date, travel, or express our sexuality, then, frequently we begin to mentally formulate a "bucket list" of what we will do when we are acceptable and are given permission to dive into new experiences. Even if we were daring non-conformists in our youth, we may have been chastised for our audacity, leaving us embarrassed and avoidant of future attempts to try new things until we are certain no one will laugh at us or admonish us for crossing the invisible line.

But, as we grow older, we tend to let go of some of our concerns about how others see us. We also suspect that – even if we manage to attain that "perfect" size or number on the scale – no matter what our age, we will never look like the models in the magazines.

There is a freedom in aging that many people write about that I didn't really believe until I turned 50. Then I truly "got it" and my new motto was, "F*#k you, I'm 50!"

I mean, really, does someone have the power to dictate what I can or cannot do because of what I look like? More importantly, why did I give others that much power over how I felt about my body for so many years? Changing that habitual way of living my life took practice, it took courage, and it took an enormous amount of, "I WILL" power. And you can do this too. And you can start now.

Why now?

Why not now? Whatever age you are, when was the last time you took an inventory of your belief system? How much of the waiting is habitual at this point? What would happen if you took a quiet moment to reflect on the things you have wanted to do in your life that you wouldn't let yourself do because of your negative body image, and see if they still interest you? Some may be outdated and no longer seductive; others may be newer additions that you were intrigued by and just assumed that you couldn't pursue until you had completed your magical transformation. As you review your waiting list, consider whose voice is telling you that those things are off limits.

Look at the situation from the present moment, in the here and now. Are the risks still as scary as they once were? Are you still willing to deprive yourself? I found that the voice telling me to wait had no real power, and I could listen to the other voice that was beseeching me to stop waiting for a time that may never present itself.

It's too bad in some ways that it took me as long as it did, but I'm certainly not going to beat myself up for not having done this sooner. I wish things in our culture were less stigmatizing and shaming towards those of us who do not fit into the narrow definition of beauty. There would be so many juicier lives being led and fewer people obsessing about such superficial matters. But, whatever age you may be, I ask you to consider walking out of the waiting room and making arrangements to fulfill some of your dreams, wishes, and goals. If it's too scary to go it alone, there may be someone who has been waiting to find someone else who was ready to stop waiting! You never know.... The important point is that you get moving ... now. Small, mindful steps are better than no steps. And remember that you, not Jenny Craig, Nutri-Systems, or Weight Watchers, are in charge of your wait management.

So ... what are you waiting for?

I hate being put "on hold." In the old days of rotary phones, if there was more than one number for the phone, there would be several plastic square buttons lined up underneath the dial. One of those buttons was red, which was the Hold Button.

As a red-haired impatient kid, when I was on a mission of whatever I perceived was of GRAND importance ... which was pretty much EVERYTHING ... being told to "please hold" was tantamount to my world screeching to a halt.

As I got older, my patience improved in many aspects of my life, but disliking being put on hold was something I never outgrew. If someone did not have the time to deal with me in that moment, then why didn't they just NOT ANSWER THE PHONE??!!

Time passed, and with it, the Hold Button morphed into the Call Waiting Click – new label ... same result. I didn't morph along with it. I was stuck in a time warp, still the impatient kid wanting to get something.

For someone who has always hated being put on hold, it is ironic how much of my life I spent putting MYSELF on hold. It was subtle at first. The weather would start getting warmer and kids would start going to the community pool or the beach. (I grew up in New York, not far from the Atlantic Ocean.) I would watch enviously as they rode off on bikes loaded with towels headed for a day of splashing and swimming. I made up excuses. "When it gets warmer, I'll go." When it got warmer, I resorted to, "I have a cold," or "I get ear aches from swimming."

Of course, the real reason was how much I dreaded having to wear a bathing suit in public. When I was unable to push the Hold Button on going, I yanked out the big gun: "I'm a redhead and I'll just get sunburned." I wore a giant t-shirt over my hideous black one-piece bathing suit, explaining when asked, "Too much sun causes skin cancer."

I tried with all of my might to stay out of sight. I put endless opportunities of having summer fun on hold because of my body-hate.

I was 9, I was 10, and on and on into my teens. I almost didn't graduate high school because of the swimming requirement in Phys. Ed.

Putting my life on hold became part of how I operated in the world:

> *When I lose weight then I will go to that party.*

When I lose weight, then I will take that class.

When I lose weight, then Davey Bernstein will like me.

When I lose weight, then I will really live the life I want to live.

How many kids are putting their lives on hold because they are being consumed by such shame and self-hate they don't give themselves the opportunity to try new things – to let go and dive in?

I think the first time I ever felt completely comfortable wearing a bathing suit was when I was pregnant and I had permission to be a fat woman in a bathing suit. The freedom I experienced was an indescribable joy. I remember that, at 8 months pregnant, I could feel my son swimming around inside of me as I was buoyantly bobbing around in the pool, completely un-self-conscious, no big t-shirt – just sunscreen and a big grin on my face.

I vowed in that moment to do three things:

The first was that – whatever traces of negative feelings I still had about my body – I would NOT push my Hold Button. I would allow my kid to experience the joys of being a kid, even if it meant wearing a bathing suit in public.

Secondly, I promised myself that whatever body shape, size, or type my child developed, I would love him unconditionally and do what I could to help him foster love and acceptance for his body.

The third and perhaps most challenging commitment was to take an active role in educating others about the damage that size discrimination can cause. Sometimes, ironically enough, this means asking people to hold their tongues and open their minds.

My son is grown now, and I am thrilled to say he has never put his life on hold, and I honestly can't remember the last time I did either.

Predictable Challenges

June introduced the concept of freedom as we began to explore our personal emancipation from our bonds of self-loathing and learning how to reject the societal constraints of fitting into a ridiculous – and for most, unattainable – standard. July expands on this as those of us who live in the U.S. face a month that opens with Independence Day.

At last, a reprieve from some of the challenges associated with body dissatisfaction and disordered eating that we have been identifying and problem solving about since January! After all, for most of us, the stressors of school are no longer in the picture, and aren't we all supposed to be enjoying the hazy-lazy-crazy days of summer?

However, what could ideally be a time for summer recreation and replenishment from academia and over-scheduled lives is an endurance test for many. It involves hiding, making excuses, covering up, and pretending. Root canals are preferred over pool parties; math homework trumps a day at the beach.

July can be a catalyst for frantic attempts to gain "body approval" before Labor Day arrives. The palpable pain of self-hate may feel intractable ... incurable. The temptation to resort to the possibility of the "quick fix" may increase, and with it, there may be a decrease in socializing and even feigning illness in order to avoid public feelings of body dissatisfaction.

It is difficult to imagine a world where summer isn't defined by our bodies, beaches, and not fitting in. Feeling like an outcast is one of the problems triggered, so connecting with places and people that provide support and encouragement is crucial. Some wonderful websites that promote positive self-image, size/self-acceptance, and de-emphasizing beauty as the primary criteria for success and happiness are:

Proud to Be Me:
PROUD2BEME.ORG

Body Positive:
FACEBOOK.COM/THEBODYPOSITIVE

We are the Real Deal:
WEARETHEREALDEAL.COM

About Face:
FACEBOOK.COM/ABOUTFACESF

With or without support systems in place, one of the goals for July is to dare to declare your independence from the societal and media messages that oppress you and steal away your love of yourself. After all, aren't we celebrating a country that guarantees all of us unalienable rights including life, liberty, and the pursuit of happiness? Those rights should apply to people of all shapes, weights, and sizes. As we enter July, we are reminded that change does not come overnight. The process of revolution and paradigm shifting may feel slow and sometimes tedious. But what about the progress you have made? What changes have you put in place since you set foot on your journey to regain a place in your heart for your body?

Important Dates to Remember

July 4th – Independence Day

Proactivity # 1

Personal Declaration of Independence

Materials

Parchment paper (or regular paper if parchment paper is not available), pen and ink, magazines, scissors and glue sticks.

–

How To

1. Think about your associations with the words life, liberty and happiness.

2. Reflect on how you may be feeling oppressed, held back, trapped, or unhappy in pursuit of living a life of liberty and happiness. Jot some of those thoughts down.

3. Put a check mark next to the restrictions that are associated with your weight or negative feelings about your body, as opposed to other barriers e.g. finances, parental permission, free time, etc.

4. Choose at least one of the areas you identified above. Using either pen/paper or cutting out words/pictures from magazines, create your own Declaration of Independence from the factors keeping you from pursuing your freedom and happiness.

5. Try to be specific so that if anyone else were to read this declaration they would know what oppression you are freeing yourself from and why.

6. Remember to sign the declaration! Feel free to make a ritual or ceremony out of the signing. Use a seal or have a witness sign it as well.

–

Why

The pressure to conform to a specific body size is rarely as oppressive as it is during the summer months when we are supposed to bare all and not have any "flaws." Frequently, when people hear the same message over and over, they begin to believe that the message is their own belief, and they stop questioning their own values. This activity provides an opportunity to identify personal values associated with life, liberty, and happiness. It is a reminder that everyone deserves these rights, and they should not be intertwined with weight, body type, or beauty. It is a powerful step to declare one's independence from an oppressor, even in such a symbolic way.

Notes

Proactivity # 2

No More Weighting

Materials

Magazines, paper, pencils, markers, personal photographs if possible.

–

How To

1. Take a moment to sit quietly and think of one thing that you have put on your "waiting to lose weight" list.

2. Using your art supplies, create a piece that shows the item on your wait list.

3. Include the obstacles that are keeping you from achieving it. Be sure to include any barriers that have nothing to do with your weight or body attitude.

4. How long has this item been on your list? Is it even something you are still interested in?

5. On a separate piece of paper, if you still desire to attain this goal, brainstorm on ways to see this through that have nothing to do with changing your body.

6. With the information you have uncovered, draw up a contract with yourself, identifying a specific plan for making this goal a reality that is not contingent on changing your body size.

–

Why

When we use our weight and body image as the primary barometers for whether or not we are allowed to do something, we put so many goals and dreams on hold. We rarely take the time to explore the endeavors deeply and see if they are possible or still desired, with or without any change in our body. In addition, when we are working on growing a healthier body image, the process can feel tedious, and we frequently forget to notice and acknowledge our progress. This activity provides the opportunity to update our wait list, acknowledge our progress, look at the list realistically, and set non-weight-related ways to move forward.

Notes

Notes

AUGUST
Project Run-away

Personal Perspectives

Have you seen them? Every August they emerge, like clockwork: the J. C. Penny ads; the Target ads; the K-Mart and Macy's ads. If you've said, "No," pat yourself on the back! Clearly you have been working on limiting your exposure to magazines and television. You are reclaiming your ability to define beauty and how much of a priority it plays in your self-acceptance.

If you are nodding your head in agreement, then you know what I am referring to:

The infamous "back to school" clothing ads.

I know, I know. While most of the country is still blistering from record heat waves and wild fires, the media is fanning our personal flames of discontent by inundating us with pictures of boys and girls and young women and men swathed in woolens, corduroys, argyles, and tweeds. According to these ads, no child is too young to "get ready" to start the new school year and "work it" with the most important back to school item of them all…

The sexiest, most flirtatious, stand-out-in-the-crowd back-to-school outfit EVER!

No doubt there is a collective sigh of relief from many as bikini season ends and is replaced, in most parts of the country, by layers of concealing sweaters. But underneath it are usually tummy-control panty hose, a constant reminder that we are still trying to compress our bodies to fit into the model of "academic babeness."

One campaign is particularly insidious and uses clothing as the ultimate weapon of "lass destruction" by pitting girls against each other based on what they are wearing. The ad assigns clothing the super power to transform a girl so completely that everyone thinks she is the "new kid" and hence gets all of the attention, leaving fallout comprised of anger and envy in the other girls. The toxic message being reinforced is girls should be more focused on being the "fairest one of all" rather than fostering healthy peer relationships and setting academic goals.

Another spot uses the classic Motown tune *Get Ready* as we watch 7- to 10-year-old girls shimmy their way into the front door of the school building. Is it a coincidence that as we get a close up of one sassy schoolgirl we hear the lyrics, "I wanna make love to you so get ready"?

Really??? Am I the only one who finds this offensive? Am I overanalyzing? Is my feminist, size-activist self, missing out on the simple joy of fashion? Am I overreacting to the K-Mart ad that has 9-year-old kids strutting down the cat walk and advising kids to "work it, girl!" (And trust me, they are NOT talking about history, science or math!)

If being outspoken on this subject and helping girls and women resist the urge to conform to the backassward priorities of our society means I come off as a Debbie Downer, then I am willing to take the heat ... literally and figuratively. It is only going to get worse between now and Labor Day. Newspapers, magazines, and internet articles will follow suit, selling fantasies of life-changing clothing with Clark Kent to Superman capabilities. And if your new clothes happen to be showing off your new body that miraculously dropped two sizes over the eight weeks you were away from your classmates, even better. What could be more amazing than showing up and hearing everyone exclaim how thin you are, enviously asking how you lost so much weight, and murmuring words of congratulations followed by hisses of "I hate you"???

You may be wondering why I care so much about this. After all, it's a tradition, a ritual, something we have all had to weather in our lifetimes... No harm. No foul. But the truth is these campaigns may spur impulsive, desperate, and dangerous last-minute attempts to drop as much weight as possible before school starts. And that is something that worries me. Additionally, as a Certified College Counselor, I am appalled at the message this sends to older students. Never mind the houses you built in Peru for Habitat for Humanity. Forget the advanced calculus classes you took at Stanford to buff up your college resume or the sacrifices you made by taking extra SAT tutoring classes. Getting your mind or your resume in shape doesn't hold an energy-saving candle to shaping up your body and wardrobe in time for the first day of school. THAT is the 4.0 that is most coveted!!!

So what can we do to prepare for this onslaught?

Plan A

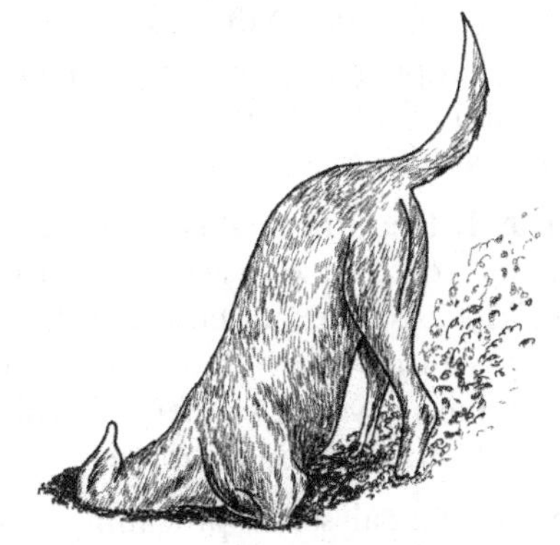

Step 1. Dig a hole

Step 2. Climb into the hole

Step 3. Stay in the hole until October.

Okay. Not realistic, and I recognize that there is a fine line between denial, avoidance, and self-preservation.

Plan B

This is a more realistic way to win the self-esteem battle and stave off the temptation to fall back into disordered eating patterns that August may trigger.

Step 1. Get Active. No, I am not talking about going on a crash exercise regimen to lose weight before the bell rings. I am talking about becoming less passive. Know what is in store for you. Prepare yourself for what you will see in the stores, magazines, on television, and on the Internet. Decide in advance how you want to control your exposure to these messages. You have more control than you think. Take an active role in what you let into your life. These media messages are aimed at selling you the notion that you are not okay in the body you have now. Would you let a friend like that into your life?

Step 2. Find your own voice and use it. You will not be able to keep all of the media messages out of your life (see Plan A) but you can neutralize the power the messages have over you. Define your own priorities for what makes a successful school year. Set your own standards for fashion, personal style, and comfort. Speak out against the media messages when possible and let people know there are more important things to focus on when the school bell rings on that first day. Attend a PTA meeting and remind parents of other ways to acknowledge their children besides weight-related measures of health and success – ones that emphasize initiative, accomplishments, and individual talents and strengths.

Step 3. Remember you are not alone. You are not the only person struggling to resist crash dieting or disordered eating when feeling vulnerable to body-appearance comparisons. Find support systems to help you maintain your resolve and reinforce your newly developing beliefs. You would be surprised how many resources are out there to help you do this. (e.g. About Face, ASDAH, Body Positive, and The Body Positive; links and information about these and other organizations can be found on my website at **drdeah.com**, or at the back of this book.)

Try to find the humor in the situation. After all, this is the month of National Clown and Smile Weeks, and without a sense of humor, it just wouldn't be funny. Be forgiving of yourself and understand that you are already a perfect size you, and no matter how much you still feel attached to changing your body, it will NOT change overnight. Hating yourself in the moment has absolutely NO positive effects on your physical or emotional health and well-being.

I remember when I was shopping for an outfit for my niece's wedding. I told myself over and over, "She is the bride. Her dress is important. Mine? Not so much." And yet, I found myself in my own personal episode of the fashion reality show, "What Not to Wear." There was an aura of importance surrounding my attire for this wedding. After all, I am the one in the family that is strident about self-acceptance. I am the one that writes a blog about redefining beauty and challenging societal standards of perfection. I am the member of the family who co-authored a book about size acceptance and women calling a truce in their battles against their bodies.

My niece was getting married. She was the bride, yet I knew I would be scrutinized. This was not narcissistic, grandiose, or ego maniacal. This was fact.

The last time I had to dress up for an important family event was for my son's Bar Mitzvah. When I was shopping for that dress, I was – "thanks" to a starvation diet – a nouveau size 4.

Step 4. I had never been that thin … and, of course, I was "just visiting." I was so inexperienced in shopping as a thin person that I accepted Saks Fifth Avenue's offer of assistance from a personal shopper.

In my typical self-deprecating way that I had cultivated over a lifetime of apologizing for my body, I looked at the personal shopper and said,

> *I'm sorry I'm such a hopeless case. It's my butt and these thighs; they must make your job so much more difficult.*

Did I mention I was a size 4? And there I was apologizing to my personal shopper for not being a size 2.

Years later, the size 4 suit that I purchased wouldn't get past my shoulders. And I no longer used a personal shopper. Flying solo, I dared to go where all too many women before me have dared to go … into the belly of the beast. Charge card in hand, I walked into The Store.

But my dress size was not the only change I had been through in the years since my son's Bar Mitzvah. I had been working on cultivating my personal size-acceptance over that time and incrementally incorporating a more Health at Every Size® (HAES®) approach into my daily routine. Hence, I was not shopping completely alone.

I entered the store with the belief that I deserved to find a dress that made me feel good. I shopped with a self-confidence that hugged my shoulders with an attitude of, "I can look just fine … beautiful, even … at this size." Most importantly, I was accompanied by my newest supportive companion: ME.

I was NOT shopping with the eyes and opinions of my family or the media. I was clad in the bullet proof vest of MY eyes and MY opinion. I was draped in a comforting serape of conviction that how I felt about how I looked and what I chose to wear was the only opinion that held any weight!!

I began looking around the store. I focused on fabrics and colors that I found pleasing. Then I included the elements of comfort and a dash of pizzazz. I was almost enjoying myself! I wasn't obsessing over what size I was or whether my arms, thighs or butt would be offensive to someone. In a way, that opened up a wider range of possibilities. True…there was still a hipper selection in the smaller single digit sizes, and that did spark my anger and caused me to write a letter of complaint to the store later that night. But I was a woman on a mission and I was not to be denied!

A saleswoman approached and I waited for my usual wave of apologetic embarrassment to wash over me. It didn't!

"That's a gorgeous dress," I said pointing towards the rack of Elie Tahari designs, "Expensive, but beautiful!"

"This dress is a classic. You will be able to wear it forever!"

I smiled when I thought of the size 4 Bar Mitzvah suit gathering dust in my closet. The personal shopper had told me the same thing, and I hadn't been convinced. After all, a part of me knew I was "just visiting" the land of size 4.

But this time I had a feeling she was absolutely correct. After years of working personally and professionally on size acceptance, my years of yo-yo dieting and shape shifting had finally come to an end!

"What size are you?" she asked, flipping through the hangers.

I smiled, and declared, "I'm a perfect size ME!"

Predictable Challenges

For a month that starts off with National Clown Week, followed by National Smile Week (I am not making this up!), one may think the "August Effect" would be one of laughter, grins, and celebration. Depending on chronological age and developmental stage, some of us are finally allowing ourselves to relax and embrace the different pace that summer brings. But for others, the sound of the clock signaling summer's end can be heard ticking louder and louder. Labor Day used to mark the end of summer, and returning to school traditionally followed that final holiday weekend. But now, many schools re-open the second or third week of August, and, depending on your point of view, you may experience a myriad of feelings including excitement, anxiety, relief, and loss.

Chin up! All is not lost! I am hoping as always, predicting the feelings associated with the upcoming changes can be a powerful proactive way to manage the "August Effect." So let's take advantage of the currents of change that are in the air all around us, and instead of being pulled down by the undertow, let's ride the wave and make some of our own intentional changes.

New beginnings may not be easy for everyone. Whether it entails going off to college for the first time, starting a new grade, re-negotiating your daily schedule back to non-summer mode, or insecurities about fitting into a new environment, we could find ourselves displacing our anxiety about transition onto body image or increase disordered eating patterns to manage these feelings. So let's take a look at turtles and snails.

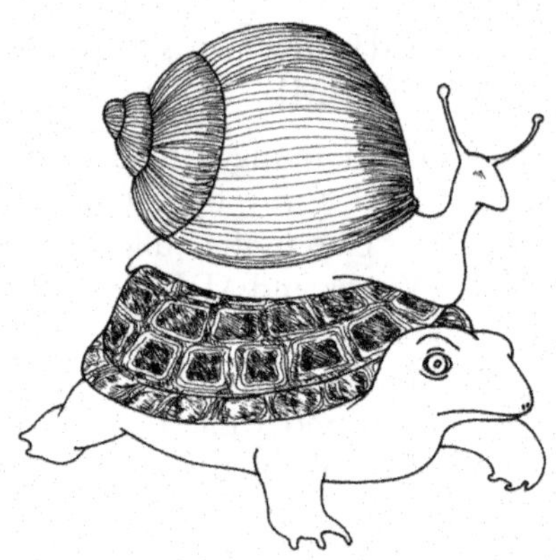

Turtles and snails??!!

I know…this is a big leap. How in the world did I go from woolen sweaters and self-actualization to turtles and snails? But bear with me for just a moment.

Turtles and snails are two creatures that carry their homes with them wherever they go. They don't change who they are based on where they are or what others expect of them. They are symbols of moving slowly and methodically – as opposed to impulsively or erratically. They know when to retreat into their shells and when to emerge. There is a tendency to equate pulling into our shells with avoidance, but there is a difference between complete avoidance and healthy self-preservation. The upcoming changes that late summer and early fall often bring do not have to mean an inevitable falling back on old habits or re-introducing negative thought processes that you may have put aside during the summer months – especially if you have a strategy to address the situation. One plan that can be helpful is- when you are making your checklist for school supplies, return-to-work task list, or dormitory linens, et cetera, take a moment and add these two items:

- What are some potential challenges that may be triggered by upcoming transitions?
- Identify a personal transitional object to bring with you.

"Transitional object?" you say. "I believe I am a bit old for a teddy bear, Dr. Deah, thank you very much!"

Okay, perhaps, but in my opinion, let's take some advice from the turtles and the snails ... we are NEVER too old for a transitional object. We may, however, need to update our definition of what a transitional object can be. Is there a word or a phrase that keeps you centered when you feel you are losing your sense of self? Is there a photo, figurine, or piece of jewelry that reminds you to breathe, focus on the positive, and stay present when you are in stressful or unfamiliar situations? Of course, human support systems are invaluable, and having someone you can call or write to is a great way to manage overwhelming feelings; but having something that is not impacted by cell phone reception or internet connectivity is more reliable. The object should be something that helps you remember your strengths and manage your anxiety. It may sound overly simplistic, a tad cheesy, and may not help at all. But in my personal and professional experience, I've seen it have positive benefits. With that in mind, let's see if we can create an adult transitional object.

Important Dates to Remember

August 1-7 – National Clown Week
Second week of August – National Smile Week
Last weekend in August – Labor Day Weekend

Proactivity # 1

Adult Transitional Object

Materials

Scissors, decoupage glue (PVA glue) and varnish, paintbrush, indelible markers, decorative paper.

Optional: Clear marble stones, printer.

–

How To

1. Take a moment and think about the metaphor of turtles and snails. These are two of many creatures that carry their homes with them wherever they go and don't lose "themselves" because they are in a new place.

2. Identify at least one positive, constant, reliable quality about yourself. If it is too hard to identify one, choose one word or one phrase that is calming or inspirational.

3. If possible, take a walk somewhere and collect smooth stones from the beach, garden, or park. This adds a pleasurable physical element to the activity. If that isn't possible, you can purchase stones or clear glass flat bottom marbles at garden stores or craft shops.

4. Hand write in marker, print out from a computer, or cut out from a magazine a word, phrase or picture that was identified in step 2 and apply to the stone or marble with decoupage glue. Allow to dry and apply several more coats for extra protection.

Optional: Add a coat of varnish on the finished product for a glossier finish.

5. Carry your object with you wherever you go.

–

Why

This is a specific application for a classic crafts activity, decoupage, or for the more recent popular craft project, inspirational stones. We tend to lose our center or our "home," if you will, when we are bombarded by media expectations of perfection or facing a life change or transition. Turtles and snails don't change who they are based on where they are or what others expect of them. This activity helps to explore and identify safe, constant, positive aspects of ourselves and create a concrete reminder (adult transitional object) we can keep with us.

Notes

Proactivity # 2

Tracings of Love

Materials

Magazines, butcher paper, construction paper, pencils, markers, scissors, glue sticks.

–

How To

1. This is an adaptation of the body tracing exercise that many art therapists use to explore discrepancies in body image.

2. Either have someone trace your body on a large piece of butcher paper, or, on the largest piece of paper you can find, draw an outline of a body. It doesn't have to be perfect. It can look like a gingerbread man!

3. On a separate piece of paper, write down the negative external messages you receive about different parts of your body.

4. Using collage materials, colors, words, and drawings, assign positive attributes to your body parts. Focus on the past and present value of those parts and what they do best.

5. Use functional adjectives like strength, motion, and specific examples. Do NOT focus on the judgments you or others have about what constitutes beauty or perfection; those thoughts and words should be written on the other piece of paper.

6. When the artwork is complete, compare the negative/critical comments with the positive ones and note the difference in how you feel based on these two different perspectives.

7. Using any kind of ritual you choose, destroy and dispose of the piece of paper with the negative thoughts and associations and keep the drawing with the positive attributes in a place where you can check it regularly.

–

Why

I usually discourage keeping fashion magazines around the house, but for this Proactivity, using magazines and other printed materials to explore body image provides a rich opportunity to acknowledge the influence of the media on our self-esteem and body acceptance. It is also a chance to assess your progress in terms of how triggering fashion magazine are in regards to your self image. In addition, this particular directive is designed to help you remember or discover that your body has more value in the world than just looking a certain way. Nurturing a true self-love for a body's abilities rather than perceived liabilities is a vital step towards living a physically and emotionally healthy lifestyle.

Notes

SEPTEMBER
Your Body or Your Life?

Personal Perspectives

I am mesmerized by the human brain. All of the classic clichés about the "wonders and miracles of nature" do not even come close to describing the remarkable capabilities of what some call our sexiest organ. My attachment to my brain is increasing exponentially as I age. This is sad, considering that my brain seems to be reveling in finding ways to let me down and disappoint me. My memory has always been one of my greatest strengths. While I could never accept a compliment about any other asset, I had no problem owning the fact that I had an unbelievable memory; and I used it professionally and personally to benefit myself, my students, and my patients. Today? It pains me to report: I live in a world of perpetual Mad Libs.

Remember Mad Libs? It was a party game where you had to fill in blanks with verbs, adjectives, nouns and the occasional gerund without knowing the context for the words. When all of the blanks were finished, the "scribe" would then read the completed version and giggles would abound at the incongruity of the words. Of course, as we got older, we made the words as sexy as possible and got very creative with four letter words … more hysterics.

Today? Not so hysterical. My brain is reMINDing me daily how hard it has been working for over half a century and is now ready for a rest and would I PLEASE not burden it with superfluous questions or concerns like:

> *What was the name of the guy in*
> *that movie with that other guy …*
> *I think they were in Texas?*

Hmmm, a proper noun … here's one. Now leave me be.

Of course, there are still memories that haunt my brain, embedded so deeply that, when accessed, I relive the experience in present time. When the memories are joyful this can be great fun. But unfortunately, my brain also holds memories of times that were so profoundly painful that, to this day, tears well up in the blink of an eye.

Some of my most negative memories revolve around my body hate and shame as a child – a common chord among those who were not the "perfect" size growing up. I still vividly remember one particular day in second grade. It was only my second time participating in the ritual, but I had already learned how to prepare for the moment when the school nurse would call, "Next…" and I would be walking the "last mile."

Unlike the walk to the "chamber" or the "chair" there was no "last meal request." In fact, I hadn't eaten since noon the previous day when the announcement over the PA warned us that "Tomorrow is weight day." That morning, I tried every trick in the book to get out of going to school, but my mother had to work, my father was already at work, and I didn't have the following pre-requisites for staying home:

- Fever over 100,
- White spots in my throat,
- An inexplicable rash.

So, reluctantly, I put on my lightest-weight clothing, even though it was winter and I was living in Far Rockaway, New York. Girls weren't allowed to wear pants to school yet, so I knew I would be cold no matter what. I might as well go ALL OUT! I went to the back of the closet where my summer clothes were hanging and pulled out the princess skirt and the light cotton blouse. "Perfect," I murmured, calculating that the combined weight of the clothing would be at least two pounds less than my warm, wonderful woolen skirt, woolen knee socks, and thick, hand-knitted, favorite gray sweater. I covered it all up with my heavy winter coat, so my mom wouldn't yell at me to change into something warmer. I threw the Cream of Wheat cereal in the garbage, and made it past her X-ray eyes. I had a higher purpose in mind. I was battling the enemy that day. It was me versus the Dark Lord, the Sith, the School Scale.

I could never understand it. Why was it so public? Why did they put the scale on the stage of the auditorium in front of everyone, while the nurse loudly announced the <u>number</u>. It was like the Salem witch trials! Why did the boys, except for Michael (name changed) NOT seem to care? Why were there other girls wearing crepe paper to school that day instead of clothing???

Why? Why? Why?

One of the first inklings I had that something was wrong with my body began when they started weighing me at school. Until then, I had been confident in my body's abilities. I played kickball, flipped baseball cards, jumped Double Dutch and was <u>no</u> slouch at Freeze Tag. I was one of the gang – that is, until I met up with Scale-a-tor, who obliterated my self-esteem in one defining moment.

"Next!" the nurse called again, impatiently. There were so many more people to humiliate, and time was ticking away. "Miss Schwartz, you are next!" I took off my shoes and socks. (Years later, when I was more into accessorizing, I would also take off my rings and watch, but that year, I was still a novice.)

"Step on." In retrospect, I wonder what would have happened if I had said, "No," curtsied and pirouetted off the stage (I also took ballet classes).

But I was obedient and stepped up. She moved the little weight bit by bit and then raised her eyebrows. She had to move the BIG weight … the one that brings you into another decade of the scale … the 10-pound weight.

I was bad.

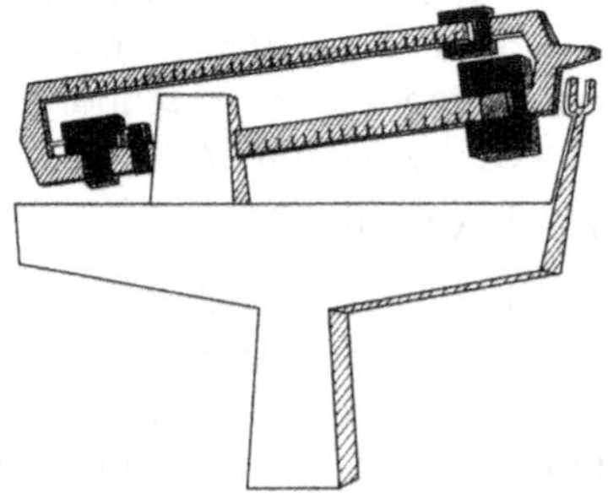

She proclaimed my weight for all to hear. I grabbed my saddle shoes, socks, and ran off the stage. I had walked the last mile, got zapped, and a part of me died.

It would take me years of personal exploration and therapy before I was able to transform my body hate into self-acceptance. Despite the decades of pain, however, I know I am one of the lucky ones. Many people reach a point where they are so tormented by the criticism and overt disgust aimed at their bodies that they end the misery by committing suicide. For those of you who think this may be far-fetched, trust me. If you had seen the number of adolescents that I worked with at a psychiatric hospital who survived suicide attempts and told me that the primary reason they wanted to die was because of how disgusting their body was, you would be less skeptical.

When I was the director of the Expressive Arts Therapy Department at a psychiatric hospital in the Bay Area, there were many ways we categorized our patients. One way was to separate the "voluntary admissions" from the "involuntary admissions." Along with the label "Voluntary Admit" was the assumption that this patient was ready to change. Conversely, the "Involuntary Admit" was being forced to change.

In both cases, change was an elusive goal; and resistance was a formidable barrier to actualizing change. Even the voluntary patients with the internal desire to change bumped up against the walls of resistance.

Change is hard. Think about it: Paper money is squishable, foldable, and malleable. Change? Metal, unyielding, rigid.

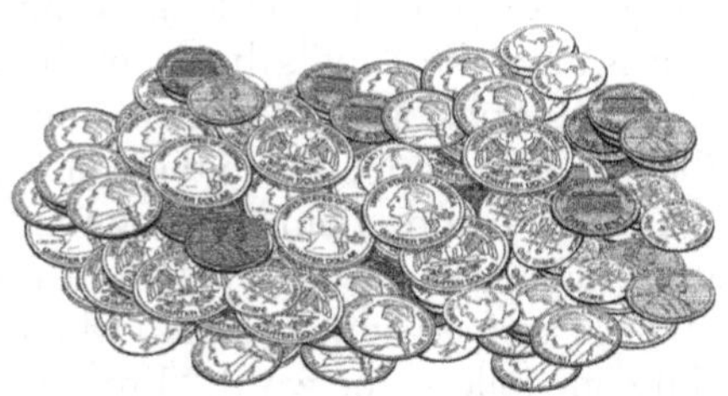

When a person embarks on the road of size-acceptance – which may or may not include changing their ways of eating or relationship with food – it is often as a result of external pressure to be different from who they are. The individual is being told over and over to change:

Change your diet.

Change your body.

Change your behavior.

Change your appearance.

The overriding message is:

You are not okay.

I worked with a patient once who told me, "If I ever kill myself, tell people it was because I couldn't stand facing another day looking in the mirror and starting the day off hating myself."

She felt like a failure every morning because she couldn't change herself into what others wanted her to be. The only definition of change she could articulate or imagine was to change the way she looked, in an attempt to please her family. Every day was an apology for her existence. Every day she put her life on hold and believed that she could only be great if she lost enough weight.

We worked on re-defining her criteria for change. We looked at why others had the authority to prescribe her "change menu." We looked at what she would change about herself if no one else had a say and she could just change what she wanted. We explored her resistance to change, from every angle.

One day in our drama therapy group she announced that she was doing a scene about the two things she wanted to change about herself more than anything.

The group waited. Would it be her butt? Her thighs? Her upper arms?

Her scene was enthralling, powerful, humorous, and poignant. As the scene ended, she was in a restaurant. She ordered her selections from the "change menu":

For my main course, I'll have the "not-giving-my-power-of-self-acceptance-away-to-my-family." And for dessert, I'll have the "learning-to-speak-Spanish-fluently," please.

It's been a while since I've heard from this patient. But from time to time I like to think of her sitting in a restaurant in Barcelona, speaking perfect Spanish and loving herself as she is. No apologies. No ifs, ands, or "butts".

And speaking of butts, I want to talk about the "But Rule."

I am really sorry, but...

I am wonderful, but...

You are totally awesome, but...

One of the rules I live by is: Be aware of what comes after the "but".

The But Rule isn't a catchy phrase or a quotable snippet like, "I before E except after C;" but, nevertheless, they are words to live by.

Here's what I mean.

Imagine a time in your life when a friend, lover, or family member, apologized to you. Chances are, the apology didn't begin and end with, "I am so sorry." Most likely the apology went more like, "I am so sorry, <u>but</u> I was really angry" or "I am so sorry, <u>but</u> you brought up the subject," or "I apologize, <u>but</u> you need to own your side of it as well."

If they had stopped at "sorry," it would have been a pure, unadulterated apology – but they didn't, because everything they said after "but" was really the message they wanted or needed you to know.

Frequently, the same holds true with compliments:

> *You look beautiful,* but *you could stand to lose a few pounds.*
>
> *She played that piece wonderfully,* but *she messed up that one arpeggio.*
>
> *He is amazing, <u>but</u> he is too short.*

And sadly, sometimes we are the violators of the But Rule. How often do we look in the mirror and say, "Great outfit, but it makes my butt look big?"

All rules have exceptions, but...

Most of the time if you look at the words after the "but", those are the true intentions of the statement, and they frequently neutralize the words that came before. I am guessing that most of us know how diluted an apology immediately becomes when someone follows the words "I'm sorry" with a justification of their mistake. In the moment, it is the apology we need, not the excuse. The excuse is usually there to convince the other person that what they did was really okay. It diffuses the apology.

Likewise, when a "but" is inserted into a compliment, the praise becomes a message of needed improvement:

> *She's great at her job, <u>but</u> she's too fat to be the face of the company.*
>
> *She's healthy, <u>but</u> she needs to lose the weight.*
>
> *He's brilliant, <u>but</u> he's fat.*

Do you see how the stigmatization of the person's body eradicates the positivity of the rest of the statement? The audience is left with the secondary image in their minds, not the first. It may seem subtle or petty, but I really believe it to be true.

As I wrote in the April chapter, despite the increasing proof of the connection between weight-bullying and suicide, few, if any, interventions are being systematically implemented in schools. Sadly, stigma is claiming more victims every day. NAAFA's End Bullying Campaign is a refreshing exception. Typically,

Anti-bullying Legislation includes protocols regarding bullying children for race, religion, and gender identity, but not for being too fat, too thin, too short, or too tall. Hence, children and adults continue to take their own lives as a result of being teased and discriminated against based on their size.

Ludicrous? Yes. Rare? No. We live in a society that gives people permission to perpetuate unapologetic hatred towards people who are, heaven forbid, fat! Read the comment sections from just about any online article or blog post about obesity, dieting, or weight management, and you will inevitably see at least one comment from someone who has no compunction about sharing their belief that:

> *FAT people deserve to die. They take up too much space and they are disgusting to look at.*

Ludicrous? Yes. Rare? No. Painful? Absolutely. Some of you may remember the 10-year-old Illinois girl who took her own life because she felt so hopeless about being fat. She is not alone. Additional studies have shown that normal-weight adolescents who merely feel fat are at risk for feelings of hopelessness, depression, and suicide.

Look, I know this is a painful and controversial topic, but the timing couldn't be more perfect to explore your thoughts and feelings on the matter. Did you know that September is National Childhood Obesity Awareness Month? The first full week in September is National Suicide Prevention Week, and the third week in September is Weight Stigma Awareness Week.

I am not sure who the people are who put together all of these awareness weeks, months, days, or years. Sometimes my linear, hungry-for-order, left side of my brain would appreciate it if they would all just come together and work from a master calendar. It would feel so much more ... well ... linear! (And this may be a primary motivation for my putting together this Calmanac). But I will say that it is not a big leap to make from Suicide Prevention Week to Weight Stigma Awareness Week. Perhaps having the two weeks so close together will prompt us to take some action, get involved, and acknowledge the need to address this preventable waste of life, whether it is in our homes, schools, workplaces, or legislatures.

For more about bullying, weight stigma, and suicide prevention, please visit these links:

- National Association to Advance Fat Acceptance (NAAFA): naafaonline.com
- Binge Eating Disorder Association (BEDA): bedaonline.com
- Association of Suicidology: suicidology.org

Predictable Challenges

Next to January, September is the month regarded as an opportunity for new beginnings.

Historically, September has been the official beginning of the new school year and a chance to start over and reinvent ourselves. We already discussed in last month's chapter the need to recognize that a new school year for children, adolescents, and college students may be fraught with insecurities about not fitting in. Bullying kids based on their body type frequently goes unchecked by adults in school. Using the justification of fighting childhood obesity (remember that September is National Childhood Obesity Awareness Month), which is being proclaimed as the new epidemic, it is becoming all too commonplace to suggest that kids as young as 4 or 5 go on restrictive diets.

This is especially disturbing, given the extensive body of research showing that these drastic attempts at weight loss often lead to eating disorders. In the spirit of a new school year and a new opportunity for learning, this is a wonderful time to review the literature, update our knowledge, and learn the facts about appropriate ways to address healthy eating and exercise habits. (Some excellent resources are available on the NAAFA website (see above) in the "Children and Parents" section) and the Association of Size Diversity and Health (ASDAH) site.

My hope is that people will stay informed on this subject and spread the word that it is time to focus on other scales to measure a child's health. We need to educate nurses, nutritionists, doctors, therapists, teachers, moms, and dads, and remind them that eating disorders among kids are escalating and directly related to self-loathing. The good news is that eating disorders and body hate are preventable, and one method is to avoid measuring a child by BMI and weight alone.

September is also frequently the month of the Jewish New Year. Because I was a "red diaper baby," I had minimal involvement with religious Jewish rituals. For those of you who are unfamiliar with the term, a "red diaper baby" is a child raised in a family that sympathized with communist/socialist tenets. In my part of the world, the New York City borough of Queens, red diaper babies were frequently the children of Atheist Jews. As a child, this meant attending Pete Seeger and Paul Robeson concerts and attending family summer camps in upstate New York or the Berkshires with names like "Camp Kinderland" and "Midvale." I attended both of these "subversive organizations" as a child, and I have fond memories of music, marshmallows, swimming, and being far, far away from the blistering heat of Far Rockaway, my hometown.

Along with the lyrics to pro-union songs, camp also taught me that there were cultural Jews and religious Jews. We were the former, and hence, my sisters and I did not miss the multitude of school days that the religious Jewish children did (BOO), nor did we have to attend religious school on the weekends (YAY).

But thrice a year we passed over the line and joined the religious Jews for Passover and the High Holidays.

My father was very clear about the reasons for these "visits" to the other side. They had less to do with God and religion and more to do with discrimination and oppression. In regards to Rosh Hashanah and Yom Kippur, the holiest of holy days, he'd explain:

> *If we were living in Nazi Germany, they wouldn't give a damn if we went to temple or not. We'd be killed just because we were born Jewish. Today you stay home from school to let everyone know that you are a Jew.*

It was an early life lesson about the irrationality of prejudice and an opportunity to watch weekday cartoons. Needless to say, we still weren't fully in the community of the "temple attending" Jews.

My grandmother, however, had both feet firmly planted in the religious Jew category, and both hands firmly planted in creating the most amazing potato knishes I have ever tasted to this day. I know I'm getting a tad sidetracked, but I need to talk about the food – the food that accompanies Jewish holidays.

The food I grew up with offered comfort, closeness, community, and cohesiveness. I don't want to talk about the calories or the confusion that amassed as I grew older resulting from being told to eat and then criticized for being fat. Mostly, I just want to reminisce with some of you and introduce others to a world of flavors and textures that filled my senses. I didn't know it then, but eating my grandma's cooking was an exercise in mindful eating, because in the world of mindful eating, it is important to really appreciate food, to relish it, to conquer ones' fear of it and to recognize satiety, hunger, and appetite.

When it came to my grandma's cooking, it was not just about my stomach being full. It was about my heart being full of her happiness that we were all together and my arms being full of loved ones and my small hands being full of dough as I helped Grandma shape the knishes. Spoons and ladles overflowed as we fed each other tastes of the proverbial Jewish grandmother chicken soup that, to borrow a metaphor from food critic Ruth Reichl, was heaven "distilled in a spoon." And her kugel, mouth-watering slippery egg noodles, buttery goodness, snuggling in between pillows of sweet pot cheese and a blanket of raisins. The top of the kugel was a comforter of crispy brown noodles. How did she get the top so crispy and keep the inside so soft, smooth, and velvety?? Miraculously there were leftovers and the next day we would eat it cold. To my delight, it was just as yummy but with a whole different array of textures on my tongue.

As we would wait for the oven to do its job, she would cut a Macintosh apple in half, scrape out one side with a teaspoon and feed me instant apple sauce … and if her apple tunnel connected to the other side of the fruit without breaking the dividing core with the seeds, I would squeal with pleasure. Then her face, usually furrowed with worries that I didn't understand, smoothed out, and was replaced with a look of satisfaction at her accomplishment.

Her knishes were flawless; the flaky pastry that my cousin Susan and I would help her prepare were filled – no, stuffed – with spicy, peppery potatoes, and the crispy top was so alluring that I would burn the top of my mouth every year because I just couldn't wait to taste one.

And then there was the tsimmis, the only dish that could transform a prune into a good time for anyone under the age of 20, and the brisket that evaporated on my tongue, if it got there (it was so tender it would often slip through the tines of the fork).

Matzoh Ball Soup. Grandma's matzoh balls would go down like a cloud but live in your stomach long enough to warrant jokes about issuing the knadlach a tenant's lease, charging it rent and giving it a name!

My grandmother had very old china, and each dish was dedicated to a specific portion of the meal. A covered bowl was the vessel for the kasha varnishkes, health food before health food was health food…who knew kasha would become a staple during my hippie days? Years later I would be living in a tipi in New Hampshire, where I was one of the only Jewish people around, cultural or religious. One day I was shopping at the co-op and I found kasha living off the radar,

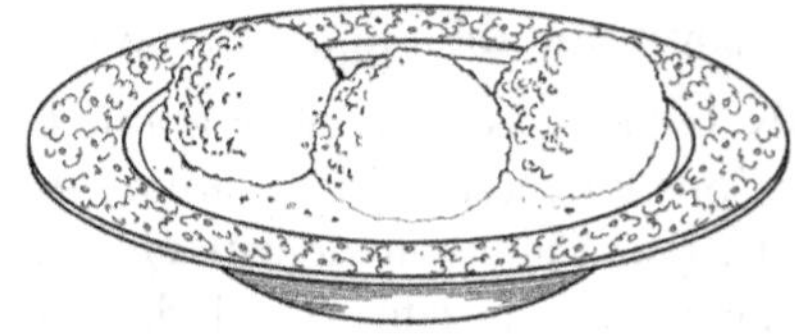

safely hiding underground under the alias of groats!

So, in September, I think about the food that accompanied my childhood years of celebrations. I find comfort in knowing that there are ways to connect with my family and other Jewish people that transcend our personal beliefs about God or our worries about calories. Instead, we sit down to a family style banquet that has to do with nurturing, and embracing our culture. I am satiated as I take in the smells, tastes, textures, memories, and company … all ingredients of the holiday food that is laid out before me. Is there any wonder that it is called comfort food?

The other tradition I have embraced from the Jewish New Year is the belief that it is time to close the book of the previous year and to begin writing your new book for the coming year. I love this metaphor – not just because I am a writer, but because it hands over the responsibility for shaping the quality of our lives to us. How we feel about our bodies is entirely in our control. How we navigate our way of eating is entirely in our hands. And how we incorporate or prioritize our personal goals of health and wellness is our personal choice.

As you will see below in the "Important Dates" section, there is an extensive list of health-related themed weeks and days. The number of these observations is indicative of this "New Year, New Start" mentality that people seem to attach to September, and is indeed, reminiscent of the New Year's resolutions from January. Whenever we are asked to observe or participate in a ritual that celebrates something, we are given a choice to accept all, part, or none of what the observance is about. This can be a wonderful opportunity to re-assess our values and beliefs, and to map out our personal itinerary for change.

The Health at Every Size (HAES®) tenets remind us that engaging in an activity that is NOT motivated by weight loss can be fun and, ultimately, result in healthier physical and emotional health. Be mindful that no one should be shamed into making choices to be healthier, and health and body size are not synonymous. Try to speak up if you feel or observe any body-shaming directed at you or someone else, even if under the auspices of good intentions and obesity prevention.

Important Dates to Remember

- First Monday of September – Labor Day
- America on the Move Month of Action: americaonthemove.org
- Healthy Aging Month: healthyaging.net
- National Childhood Obesity Awareness Month: fitness.gov
- National Yoga Month: yogamonth.org
- First week of September – Suicide Prevention Week: suicidology.org
- Third week of September – National Weight Stigma Awareness Week: bedaonline.com
- Last full week of September – Active Aging Week: icaa.cc
- September 21 – International Day of Peace: un.org/en/events/peaceday
- September 22 – First day of fall
- Last Wednesday of September – International Women's Health and Fitness Day: fitnessday.com/women
- Last Saturday of September – Family Health and Fitness Day: fitnessday.com/family

First Monday of September – Labor Day
September 21 – International Day of Peace, un.org/en/events/peaceday

Proactivity # 1

Mapping Out Change

Materials

Large sheet of drawing paper, markers or colored pencils. Optional: magazines, scissors, glue sticks.

–

How To

1. Make a list of changes that are coming down the road in September.

2. Color code them in terms of difficulty, with red being the hardest and blue being the easiest adjustments to make.

3. Using your art materials and your creativity, draw a road map similar to a road trip itinerary with each change being a "stop" along the route. Remember to incorporate the color coding so you can see where you are predicting the road will have a speed bump or pothole.

4. When your map is finished, brainstorm about the road side assistance or services that may help you manage the changes. Show them on the map as well. For example, on a road trip it is important to know where you can get gas or meals along the way; or where to build in a rest stop or a time for some scenic viewing. Carefully include your support systems and coping mechanisms on the map near the places you are anticipating less-than-smooth sailing.

–

Why

September is an opportunity to look at what your upcoming journey for the next several months look like, and the analogy of a road map helps to view change as just another part of life's journey. Predicting events and potential potholes helps to instill a sense of control over the circumstances that lie ahead and to identify effective and non-self-destructive ways to either navigate around or repair them.

Notes

Notes

Proactivity # 2

Put Out That But!

Materials

A small notebook and a pencil or pen.

–

How To

1. Throughout the week, pay attention to how you and others use the word "but" and see if you notice The But Rule. Remember, The But Rule is: When we make an apology or a positive statement there are often two sections to the statement: pre- and post-but. The words after "but" frequently diffuse the apology, or, when used in conjunction with a compliment, transform simple praise into an objective or goal for improvement.

2. Jot down as many examples as you can. Try to be specific about the events surrounding the incident. Also note the following: How is the person you are speaking with (or yourself) reacting to what is being said? What is the impact on your self-esteem when you qualify your positive self-statements with a post-but statement? How does it change the effectiveness or authenticity of the communication?

3. At the end of the week, review the entries and see if you can find a pattern in these interactions. Are the same people involved? Is the subject matter the same each time? Were you able to see or feel the result on your self-esteem when the But Rule occurred?

4. Now, choose at least one event and rewrite the scenario using different language to express the same sentiment this time NOT using the word "but." Does this feel different at all? If so, why? If not, why not?

–

Why

The third week of September is Weight Stigma Awareness Week. This activity increases our awareness of how we may unconsciously put ourselves down and sabotage building a positive body image. It allows us to practice using new language and perhaps let others know how they could be using a more body-positive form of communication.

Notes

OCTOBER
I Love My Body, I Love My Body!

Personal Perspectives

If you have been reading this book from the beginning, you may have noticed by now that there is a day for everything!!! I kid you not. March 14th is National Potato Chip Day, November 7th is Bittersweet Chocolate with Almonds Day, and my personal fave – that happens to fall on my birthday, December 13th – National Ice Cream Day!

There are, however, dedicated days and weeks that I take more seriously, and they are steadily increasing year after year. In fact, I need a calendar to keep track of all of the special dates that pertain to a body positive approach to wellness. Of course, I wish we didn't need any of these days, weeks or months. Because when you really examine them, it is a sad state of affairs that we need to be reminded to:

- Love your body (Third Wednesday of October)
- Reject diets (May 6th)
- Prevent Eating Disorders (February 20-26)
- Adopt the ideology of Healthy Weight Awareness (third week of January)

But for now, let's take a look at Love Your Body Day. Does this day mean I should love your body? Or, does it mean I should love my body? As Bugs Bunny would say, "Ain't language a stinkuh?" I am in love with language. If I could choose one superpower, it would be fluency in every language. I would have the ultimate zoo key that would allow me to communicate with people in every culture.

Remember zoo keys? They were plastic keys, usually in the shape of an elephant, that were inserted in "talking boxes" around the zoo. When you turned the key, a voice inside the box would tell you all about the animal. Without the key, you only had your eyes and perhaps your teacher's or parent's limited knowledge about the koala. But with the key, you knew the koala's name was Kool Hand Koala, his country of origin, and that he had the hots

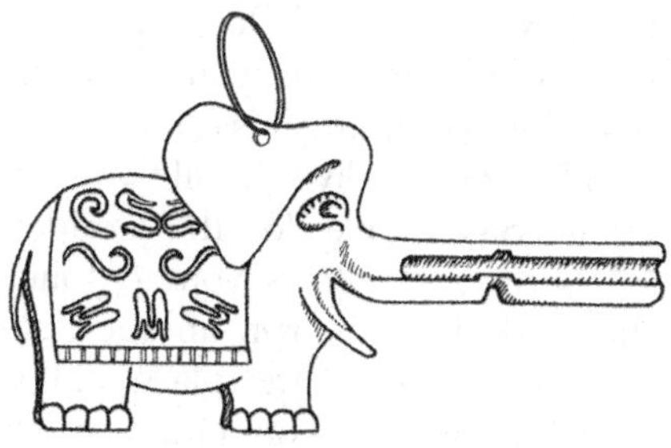

for his cage mate, the lovely and Kurvaceous Koolata. The mystery of the koala was solved thanks to the special plastic key that only some people were fortunate enough to own – assuming, of course, they knew English.

But my love of language isn't confined to the spoken word. It extends to the written word, which has its own nuances and delightful mysteries that can be wonderful and pesky! For years when I was reading the name Hermione in the Harry Potter books, in my head I heard "Her-me-own." My own name commands the same response from many people. When a reader sees my name written, Deah, they hear in their heads, "Dee-uh". It is in fact Day-(like the opposite of night) uh. Once someone knows my name, when they see it written, they can hear it in their heads as Day-uh as I now hear "Her-miney."

These discrepancies inherent in "written pronunciation" are also, unfortunately, the cause of many arguments in the worlds of blogs and e-mail. How many of us have gotten into arguments because what we wrote is not read with the lilt in our voice and twinkle in our eye that was there when we hit the "send" button? Written language as a medium can be painfully one-dimensional, and it takes a true wordsmith to effectively convey sarcasm, empathy, and gentleness through their writing. Processing disagreements should never be addressed via e-mail for just this reason, and writing a blog on controversial topics demands hyper-vigilance if one doesn't want to be misinterpreted and potentially alienate their readers.

But auditory double entendres can also be delightful to play with. For example:

> *I really hope you pull this off.*

Or,

> *You are the last person he wanted to see.*

Depending on the context of these statements they can have totally different meanings ranging from hurtful and rude to sexy and logistical. "I hope you pull this off" can be supportive or brashly seductive. "The last person he wanted to see" is fine if a doctor is scheduling an appointment with you, but not so great if the doctor is saying they don't want to see you ever … at all! I know there are people out there who insist that words are "just words" and shouldn't make such an impact. But are they just words … as in, words of justice or fairness? Or just words as in merely or simply? Either way, thankfully, there are enough people who take words seriously and understand that the context of words is vital for understanding their intended meanings.

There are those special times when either interpretation can be positive. If someone writes me a note and tells me, "I just read your blog," this could mean that my blog is the ONLY blog they read, or that they just finished reading my latest post. Both are really good news. I love when that happens.

So let's take a look at the upcoming Love Your Body Day. Some read this and believe it is a directive to love their own body:

I love my body I love my body!

Today is the day that I "love my body!" Others interpret it that they should love someone else's body:

I love your body, I love your body!

Today is the day to acknowledge that "I love your body!"

Either interpretation, in this case, reminds us to take a day (which really should be every day) to respect and appreciate the diversity of our own and each other's bodies and NOT give in to the prevalent message that is fed to us every day: that unless our bodies conform to a homogenous standard, they do not deserve our love.

So, until there is a paradigm change and we mark on our calendars that every day is Love Ourselves Day, bodies and all, let's celebrate the third Wednesday of October. Spend the day appreciating your amazing body for everything it is doing, 24/7, to allow you to live the life you are living. Say thanks for the wonderful body that allows you to touch the world in your own unique fashion, making it a better place. Then when you wake up on Thursday, try it again, and the next day, and the next day.

Another big day in October is Halloween. If I had to describe my relationship with Halloween in Facebook lingo I would have to choose "it's complicated," and I am sure I am not the only one.

Halloween could have been my favorite holiday. It had all the makings for the Perfect Good Time: Running around dressed up as anything or anyone you wanted, collecting and eating massive amounts of candy, not having to sit through some long drawn out ritual or service before being allowed to run around at night, (collecting and eating massive amounts of candy). And let's not forget the lovely after-glow of the candy lingering in the house … sometimes for as long as a week. That made the eight days of Chanukah pale in comparison.

It was also the perfect inter-generational holiday. There was no age limit to participate. You were either the giver or receiver, and dressing up was allowed no matter what age you were … except for those two pesky years of adolescence when you felt it was totally uncool to dress up. But even then, no one said you couldn't. It was your choice. I remember, during my "trick or tweening" years, feeling a little sorry for the kids who still had to trick or treat with their parents. Decades later, as a mom, I learned that despite the kid's possible discomfort, the parents were relishing in the few years we were allowed to accompany them! And that was a treat! We were all grown up but gallivanting from house to house, anonymously clad in costume, and reliving the hedonistic pleasure of taking over the night and hauling in massive amounts of free candy. Why do you think we call it "Haul"oween?

I was born in Queens and then moved to the 'burbs of Long Island. In contemplating the ultimate Halloween question, "Which is better, city or suburb trick or treating?" If quantity is the barometer for a successful Halloween, then trick or treating in apartment buildings in New York is the indisputable victor! Imagine floor after floor and door after door ... lined up ... each handing out candy. It was a one-stop-shop candy jackpot: most amount of candy, least amount of effort.

The suburbs, on the other hand, made you work harder for your treats ... trudging from house to house, up looong driveways, climbing stairways to giant web-laced doors-just to get pennies for UNICEF and apples with razor blades (just kidding about the apples; but for some reason, it wasn't until I moved to the 'burbs that I heard stories of tainted treats). But there were still massive amounts of free candy. Granted, you had to cover more ground to get the same amount of candy that you got in the city, but the candy was dandy nonetheless, and the neighborhood streets were swarming with kids who had been waiting for dusk since school let out at 3:00p.m. (Because the unwritten rule was that you couldn't start trick or treating until it was dark).

Once in a while you'd ring a bell and a wise guy (usually a dad) would open the door dressed as a monster. We'd squeal with delight and yell in unison, "Trick or treat," and with a twinkle in his ghoulish eye he'd say, "Trick."

We would freeze ... not knowing really what that meant ... or what we were supposed to do ... and just as it started to get tense, the Grim Reaper would grin a self-satisfied smile, put down his plastic scythe, and dole out handfuls of candy corn and bite-sized Snickers.

How could this not be a great holiday?

And it was...until around fourth grade, when my trick-or-treating days changed forever.

Food became my enemy and candy the Darth Vader of my universe. As I mentioned in a previous chapter, in my household, at any given time, my mother, father, or the kids were on diets. This, of course, meant no treats in our house or in our mouths. As I was indoctrinated into the lifestyle of weight cycling diets in the attempt to please those around me with a thin, lithe body, Halloween became the perfect opportunity for a binge. Better yet, it was sanctified by all of the Powers That Be. Passover Shmassover … THIS was the holiday that begged me to question:

> *Why is this night different from all other nights???*

And the answer,

> *Because on this night you can collect and eat all of the candy you want!*

The TV showed it, the movies showed it, the magazines wrote about it, let's face it … it was National Annual Binge on Candy Day!

And it terrified me.

More than any haunted house, more than any midnight showing of *Night of the Living Dead*, even more than the Kappa Delta Nu "gang" waiting in the shadows to pummel us with eggs: The scariest part of Halloween for me was the candy. For years I woke up the morning after, like an alcoholic waking from a bar-hopping spree – incredulous at the amount of candy wrappers surrounding me and the weight of guilt I had gained by engaging in the simple pleasure of Halloween. I found it hard to fathom why my friends' candy would last for weeks and weeks, eventually becoming too stale and hard for their braces, at which point it would be unceremoniously tossed. Mine was gone within a week.

The treats were no longer treats.

And then, just when I thought it couldn't get any worse, it did.

In my early teens I became aware of a whole new trend in dressing up. All of sudden, there were costumes being advertised, that somehow in my pre-

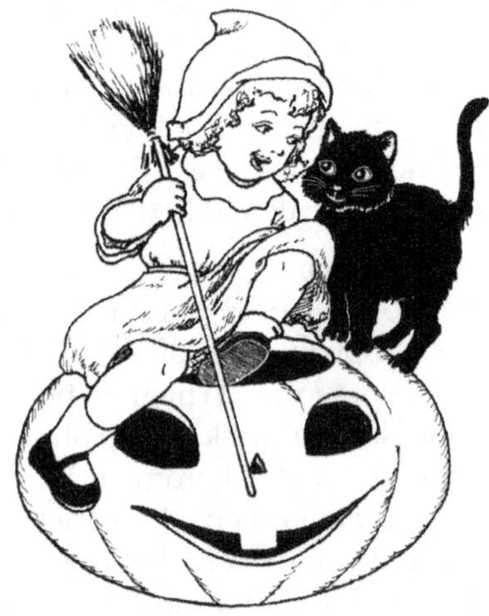

pubescent naiveté I hadn't noticed before. They were the same costumes I had always seen: the black cats, Wonder Woman, Bat Girl, belly dancer, nurse, only now they were <u>sexy</u> … seductive … flesh revealing and titillating. Next to ads with centerfolds of mini Mounds bars and candy corn were centerfolds of young girls with mini mounds protruding out of their Xena Warrior Woman costumes.

New questions were formulating in my brain. How could I be expected to gorge on candy and fit into a skimpy costume? When did Halloween become about my body? And under my anger was a longing to fit in. I yearned for the days when I could dress up for the fun of it and not worry if I looked good or pretty or sexy in my costume.

Please don't get me wrong. I am not a prude about sexuality. But seeing 13-year-olds dressed up as sex-pot Tinkerbells just … well … disturbs me. Now, when the Grim Reaper opens the door and responds to the chorus of "Trick or treat!" with, "Trick!" I can't stop my brain from thinking "brothel."

So, what's a mother to do? Because so many of us regard chocolate and candy in general as forbidden food, when a holiday like Halloween comes along, it may be difficult to maintain our ghoul … um … cool. Many parents have rules about what their kids can do with their candy. Some allow the kids to eat as much as they want for that night and then the rest gets thrown away. Others dole it out one or two pieces a day for seven days or until it's gone. I understand a parent's intention to set limits and help kids establish healthy food habits, but care needs to be taken as to how this is done. Presenting candy as the enemy (assuming there are no allergies or medical conditions to take into consideration) may lead to sneak eating or an all-out binge. Sometimes these eating patterns get generalized to other holidays, events, and meals, ultimately developing into more complicated disordered eating behaviors.

It is important to teach kids about mindful eating early on, resisting the temptation to introduce restrictive diets that label foods as "good" food or "bad" food. I remember when I was 16 and realized that those mini-candies were available all year long! That was the last time I binged on them on Halloween. Knowing I didn't have to eat them all in one night or the few days that followed (because it would be another YEAR before I could eat them again) diffused the compulsion and drove a wooden stake into Count Chocula's heart. If candy is not an evil food that shows up once a year like the Jason movies, then the urge to binge is lessened and the fun is in the collecting and the dressing up, not in the consuming.

The part about why little girls have to dress up in sexually provocative costumes, I haven't figured out yet. In 2008, a costume called "Anna Rexia" hit the shelves. It was a skeleton costume designed to expose as much cleavage and skin as possible. There was an outcry of rage. Some stores listened and removed the costume from the shelves.

In the late 1970s, I had a job at a preschool program in Marin, California. It was my first time working with kids that young, and I was excited to add that age group to my repertoire. The kids were totally adorable and wide open to trying all of my theater, art, movement, and recreational activities. The lack of inhibition was so refreshing, especially compared to the adolescent population I had worked with at my last job.

These 3- to 5-year-old children, in retrospect, reminded me of that greeting card that was so popular a few years ago. It went something like, "Dance as if no one is looking, sing as if no one is listening…" et cetera. They were fearless, spontaneous and trusting. With one exception.

During the course of the school day there was a designated free-play time. Stations were set up around the classroom and the kids could choose an activity at any of the stations. Free play was justified by the staff as age appropriate, designed to foster decision-making skills, and to improve social interaction and leisure awareness. And it was supposed to be fun! One of the stations was a dress up corner overflowing with an extensive array of costumes, props and a few mirrors for admiring outfits.

My personal memories of dressing up as a little kid were wonderful, especially in juxtaposition to my later years of torment in real-life dressing rooms, like those furtive, embarrassing visits to Lane Bryant in order to find something that would fit. As a 3- to 5-year-old kid, I savored the opportunities at my preschool to transform into a pirate, cowgirl, and, of course, the ultimate dress-up op: a princess. It WAS fun!

The first time I heard Jenny (not her real name) say, "No" to an invitation to play dress up, I didn't pay much attention. She had been completely absorbed, in that tongue-out-of-the-mouth, completely focused way that preschoolers have, with a Play-Doh machine. Squishing the red dough out in spaghetti strands, the blue dough out in long fat cylinders, and squealing with delight as the green dough emerged in heart shaped noodles, she probably would have said, "No!" to pony rides in that moment – or so I thought.

As the weeks passed, however, I noticed that the only station she NEVER visited was the dress-up corner, even though from time to time I would see her sneaking glimpses of the other kids as they danced around with an abandon that would have put Salomé to shame. After a few weeks, the other kids stopped asking her to join them in rifling through the trunks and racks of clothing: It was understood that Jenny just did not "do dress up."

If Jenny had been a noticeably "overweight" kid, I may have had some clue as to the reason behind her reluctance. But Jenny was a solid, athletic, and active child; so if it hadn't been for our end-of-the-year production for the parents, I never would have known the why.

We were getting ready for our extravaganza, and all of the kids were putting on their hats, funny noses, boas, feathers, and costumes. Jenny was standing off to the side, fussing with a witch's dress … tugging and pulling … frowning … forehead knitted. I came up next to her with a hat for her outfit.

She looked at me as she took the hat and said, "Am I fat in this dress?"

My heart sank. This had been her reason all of these months for avoiding the dress-up corner, and now it was wheedling in on her ability to enjoy the end-of-the-year showcase! There was so much I wanted to say, starting with,

> *Even if the dress did make you look fat, why is that bad?*

Or,

> *Is this what you see your mom do when she is getting dressed in front of the mirror?*

Or,

> *Yes, you look like a big fat fabulous witch, woo hoo!*

But I just looked into her 5-year-old eyes, knowing that this was one of those teachable moments and not knowing what to say. I was, if you can imagine, speechless.

I turned her away from the mirror, zipped up the dress, put the hat on her head and as I began painting her face green I said,

> *That dress makes you look like a scary witch! You are perfect. Now let's practice your cackle!!*

Predictable Challenges

Halloween is a tricky holiday for people struggling with body dissatisfaction and eating disorders. The ritual of trick-or-treating, whether you are on the giving or collecting side, can be fraught with frights that morph miniature chocolate bars into chainsaw-wielding serial killers. In addition, the preoccupation with consuming is magnified by the emphasis on costuming. Dressing up for Halloween adds another layer of anxiety and despair for those who may want to join in the fun but feel that the availability of costumes in larger sizes is limited – not only in terms of where they can be purchased, but the breadth of choices that are deemed "fat friendly."

The secret and mysterious nature of Halloween is replicated in how secretive many people are about their disordered eating and body dissatisfaction. Choosing to mask instead of share feelings is common and results in silent suffering and clandestine binge-eating episodes to manage the stress.

Fortunately, Halloween is at the end of the month, which provides 3 to 4 weeks to proactively prepare to navigate this ghoulish time of the year.

Here are some things to consider: Are you masking or hiding your feelings with:

- Restrictive dieting or binge eating?
- Obsessing about your weight?

• Engaging in negative body talk either by yourself or with others?

When you think about Halloween:

• Do you feel anxious about the availability of Halloween candy?

• Are you limiting your participation in fun events due to not feeling thin enough to wear a costume or "strong" enough to resist the treats?

Take some time to explore what may happen if you:

• Declared a truce with yourself this Halloween and gave yourself permission to accept your body at the size it is now.

• Experiment with the idea that there are no "good" or "bad" foods (as long as there are no allergies or medical problems associated with specific foods) and that Halloween candy is available all year long.

• Do you think you would still binge if you trusted the fact that this is not your ONLY chance to have these treats?

Important Dates to Remember

• Eat Better Eat Together Month: wsu.edu/ebet

• Children's Health Month: yosemite.epa.gov/ochp/ochpweb/nsf/content/chm-home.htm

• Breast Cancer Awareness Month: nbcam.org

• National Depression and Mental Health Screening Month: mentalhealthscreening.org

• First Monday in October – Child's Health Day: mchb.hrsa.gov

• October 10 – World Mental Health Day: wfmh.org

• Third Wednesday in October – Love your Body Day: loveyourbody.nowfoundation.org

• Third week in October – National Health Education Week AND National Healthcare Quality Week: nahq.org

• October 31 – Halloween

All month – National Depression and Mental Health Screening Month, mentalhealthscreening.org
Third Wednesday in October – Love your Body Day, loveyourbody.nowfoundation.org
October 31 – Halloween

Proactivity # 1

Unmasked

Masks can be created in a variety of ways depending on your budget and how much time you would like to devote to the process. For example, if time is an issue, already-made blank masks can be purchased and decorated using paints, markers, fabric, stickers, et cetera. With more time you can create the mask out of papier-mâché or plaster cast strips and then decorate it. Here is how to create a mask using plaster strips.

–

Materials

Plaster cast strips (they can be found in school or medical supply stores – you'll need one roll per mask), bowl of warm water, Vaseline, scissors, string (if you want to wear the mask for role plays or hang the mask up), materials for decorating the finished mask – e.g., glue fabric, buttons, photographs, paint, et cetera, drawing paper and markers, pencils, pens, or crayons.

Optional: Hair covering (headband or shower cap), rubber gloves, and/or smock to protect hands and clothing (this can be a messy activity).

–

How To

1. Cut plaster tape into pieces of varying lengths. It is important to keep strips dry until used so the plaster doesn't harden.

2. Pull back hair and apply a light coat of Vaseline on forehead and around the area where the mask is going to be made.

3. Dip the plaster strips in the water and apply them to the face, making sure that the side of the tape with the extra plaster is facing out. Repeat this step three times using extra tape around the bridge of the nose; then let dry for about 15 minutes.

4. Carefully remove the mask and let dry for 24 hours.

5. While the mask is drying, take some time to think and free write about what you mask with your body hate and disordered eating and why. If your attention wasn't constantly tied up with weight and body image issues, what other aspects of yourself would be revealed?

6. Now, think about what your mask would look like if it represented either:

A. An aspect of yourself that is being suppressed, avoided, or undiscovered.

B. A new coping strategy other than food or body preoccupation to help deal with difficult feelings and life challenges.

C. A fear or fantasy of what would happen if you discarded your food and/or body preoccupation.

7. On a separate piece of paper, using pencils, markers, crayons, et cetera, plan what your mask will look like.

8. Using the art supplies available, create your mask.

Why

Wearing a mask in our society is typically associated with costume parties and Halloween. We often select masks in order to try on other personas that are different from our day-to-day personalities.

This expressive arts therapy directive asks you to make a mask that represents a part of you which is typically masked by eating patterns and/or body dissatisfaction, so that you can address your fears and fantasies of what would happen if you discarded these preoccupations.

Notes

Notes

Heal-o-ween

Materials

Paper, scissors, glue sticks, markers, magazines or other collage materials.

–

How To

1. Take a moment and sit quietly. Imagine you are able to push a button and magically lose all of your body hate without your body weight changing one iota.

2. What fears come to mind when you entertain that possibility? What are you afraid you will lose along with the hate? What are you afraid you will have to do differently if you lost the hate? Will people treat you differently? Will you have to act differently? Be specific and remember this is just a "scary movie." None of it is REALLY HAPPENING! It is Halloween!

3. Using your art supplies, create either a film story board depicting at least one of the scenarios as if it is a scene from a horror movie, or make a collage of the fears. No one else has to see this, so be as creative and honest as possible.

4. When your piece is complete, look at it closely. How probable is it that these fears will happen in real life? Are they powerful enough to keep you from exploring a more positive relationship with your body? Are there other possibilities, less frightening, that you haven't considered?

5. On a separate piece of paper, create a new, less frightening, less Hollywood-esque scenario that could also be a possibility if you chose to push the Lose Body Hate Button.

–

Why

Halloween is all about things that are spooky, scary, eerie, creepy. Losing our body hate is difficult for many of us because we are afraid of what will happen if we let go of hating our bodies and choose body love and self-acceptance instead. This activity gives us a safe, non-judgmental space to explore what we are afraid of and then to objectively assess whether those fears are grounded in reality. It also provides the chance to brainstorm on whether or not we are open to trying a new course of action, and if so, what that would be?

Notes

Notes

NOVEMBER
Thank Yourself

Personal Perspectives

Thanksgiving is a difficult holiday for me. There is no doubt that part of my ambivalence about Thanksgiving stems from my childhood. Up until I was 12, Thanksgiving was all about going to the New York City Macy's Day Parade, followed by a dinner where we were allowed to eat our favorite foods with abandon. The usual scrutiny and admonishment for eating a full meal, instead of the typical array of carefully measured-out diet foods, was suspended for the Thanksgiving feast. In its place we were given a "blank check" which was good for an unlimited amount of talking about the meal, preparing the meal, eating the meal, eating more of the meal, eating the leftovers, and, without a teaspoon of self-consciousness, rolling off of our chairs at the end of the meal comparing our "stuffitudeness."

We all intentionally wore our comfortable baggier clothing on Thanksgiving in preparation for the feast. Thanksgiving Day – perhaps more than any other holiday – was about what was good in the world, what was working, what was right.

Then everything changed.

In 1969, one month before my 13th birthday, we went to the parade as usual, but afterward we went to visit my mom, who was in the hospital. I hadn't seen her since October when she was admitted, because hospitals back then were very strict about kids being on the unit and getting in the way. I gingerly perched on the edge of her bed and we talked about the infamous gigantic parade balloons. She asked me to describe which were my favorites this year, which weren't, and if I saw any famous people on the floats. Of course, I had no idea this would be the last time I would see my mom alive. As I hugged her goodbye, careful not to disturb any of the tubes, I was anxious to leave this imposing hospital room with the strange sounds and smells that I didn't associate with my mom at all. When I was finally back on the street, I breathed a sigh of relief and just assumed that my mom would be home very soon.

I don't remember what we did for our Thanksgiving meal that day. Whatever it was, the food and celebration were eclipsed by the experience at New York Hospital, one I was eager to forget. This doesn't mean that I never enjoyed another Thanksgiving again after that, but it did give me a taste of the reality that any given holiday is NOT a holiday for everyone. I became aware of certain generalized assumptions that are made about how people are supposed to feel and behave around holidays. The darker underbelly of the holidays is often not addressed, and many people may feel worse because they can't rally and get into the holiday spirit when the demands to be jovial are coming from all around them. But when people are given permission to voice their ambivalence about the pressure to act celebratory, and to explore and express both the holiday blues and the holiday glees, the result is inherently therapeutic. After all, holidays can bring back memories of being with people who have passed or, like in my situation, may be anniversaries of times that were not filled with quite so much holiday cheer.

Additional reasons that Thanksgiving may be problematic for some folks include: politics, Native American issues, protests of vegetarians on behalf of the ritual menus, obligatory visits with family members that may not be entirely comfortable, and having to look a certain way to join in on the festivities. Then of course, if there are any eating disorder issues, feast-centric holidays frequently exacerbate those challenges.

So, what is the perfect recipe for a perfect Thanksgiving celebration?

I am so glad you asked! Here are six of my favorite tried-and-true recommendations:

1.

Remove the word "perfect" from the equation. Oftentimes, the focus of Thanksgiving is predominantly on serving the perfect meal on the perfectly set table and being the perfect host/hostess. Try to relax and remember that almost everyone who is sitting at your table is already at least 94% thrilled that you are taking on the work of the Thanksgiving feast and that they didn't have to!

2.

Remember that this is just another dinner. When I gave up on dieting, I realized that I could have Thanksgiving favorite foods all year long, and because I wasn't living in a constant state of deprivation through dieting, I knew that I didn't have to eat an exaggerated amount of sweet potato marshmallow casserole or sausage stuffing. I could eat this meal like any other meal, savor the flavors and understand that the success of the event was not measured by how far into a food coma I would find myself.

Today, I always put aside leftovers so that I don't activate that Binge Eating Disorder (BED) part of me that defiantly needs to binge proactively because I fear not having access to that wonderful food ever again. The food is only part of the party–not the whole kit and kaboodle.

3.

Honor the diversity of people's associations with the occasion. Usually, Thanksgiving has some kind of ritual that involves each person saying something they feel grateful for. In order to lessen the pressure to squelch feelings or risk being labeled as negative or non-participatory, offer the option of an open-ended question. For example:

> *What does Thanksgiving mean to you?*

Or,

> *If you could add anything to the celebration of Thanksgiving, what would it be?*

4.

Include generous amounts of humor, cook with joy, and acknowledge our fabulous miraculous bodies for what they CAN do and do not negate or hate them because of what they look like. No matter what your opinion is of the reason for getting together to celebrate this holiday-it offers us an opportunity to take a moment out of our busy lives, to appreciate some of the wonderful acts of kindness and grace that we bestow on ourselves, and others. We get to acknowledge the goodness that has come our way. Add a few cups of unconditional loving, a bowl of self-acceptance, and you have the fixings for a luscious and meaningful Thanksgiving.

5.

Lose the Guilt! There is no time like the present to start Dr. Deah's Guilt-Free Diet!

Yes, you read that correctly. I am promoting a restrictive diet and I am inviting you to join me in my Guilt-Loss Program. One of the comments I hear frequently in my work is some version of:

> *I really want to embrace the Health at Every Size point of view. In fact, I do embrace it. I live it, I breathe it, and I believe in it. But I'm still attached to wanting to be thin. I feel guilty about that. Do you still like me? Can I still be a part of your club? Am I okay???*

The answer is:

> *Yes. You are human.*

I know it's hard to believe that there is a point of view where you can define your own standard of beauty that takes into consideration your body's natural shape and is NOT based on comparisons or someone else capitalizing on your feeling that you are not ENOUGH.

And your skepticism makes sense because there is a paucity of places in our lives where we are allowed to just "be enough." Even places we assume to be guilt-free safe havens turn out to be hot beds of comparisons, insecurity, and feeling guilty about not "doing it right."

Take yoga, for example. I used to take yoga. I lived on an ashram and everything. It was the most competitive environment I had ever been in! My poses weren't "posey" enough, my gauzy drawstring pants weren't gauzy enough, and my mat was a towel. We were supposed to be going inward as we went downward dog; but a quick glance sideways inevitably revealed that everyone was looking at each other to see if they were stretching as far as the person next to them. I don't want to digress and have people think I don't love yoga. I do. And now there are yoga classes for people of all sizes proliferating around the country. (I have a list of Size Diverse Yoga Classes in the resource section of my website under "Yoga Professionals"). But for me, when yoga turned into X-TREME ASS-ANAS with the heat cranked up to 90+ degrees and the sun salutation was done in fast forward with techno music blasting … well let's just say I didn't want to be Jane F*#*ing Fondananda and feel the Bikram Burn. (I don't judge anyone that enjoys the Bikram method. It's just NOT for me.) It got in my way of reaping the benefits of a more gentle practice and exacerbated my tendency to feel excluded and guilty that I wasn't doing it fast enough.

So enough with the guilt already! I chose to find a more ego-syntonic movement and I found that HAES fit the bill for me.

- An inclusive movement means just that: INCLUSIVE! A size-acceptance movement means just that: ALL sizes accepted.
- A self-acceptance movement means that our goal is to accept ourselves and each other at any size.
- This does not mean you have to stay fat.
- This does not mean you have to love every minute of being fat.
- This does not mean you have to stay thin.
- This does not mean that you don't have personal preferences.
- This does not mean that you don't wish you could fit into your pre-menopausal-weight-gain clothing because you don't have enough money to buy new clothes because you have to pay for your expenses to go to a conference and sell your book so you will have money to buy new clothes …(Oooh, see how I made that all about me??)
- It especially does <u>not</u> mean that you should be bullied or ostraSIZED for being whatever size you are.

Seriously, how much happier would we be if we just lost The Guilt? We weren't born with The Guilt. We can survive without The Guilt. It is not a primal instinct. It doesn't feed us, clothe us, keep us safe, and it certainly does not make us happy.

Guilt is NOT the same as remorse.

Someone who is able to feel badly about hurting another living being or committing a cruel act against society is showing that they have a conscience. They can tell right from wrong and hopefully learn from the experience and change. Remorse and empathy can be liberating. Guilt? Guilt just festers. It's like a black mold that begets more and more black mold until you are completely filled with guilt and feel like a failure.

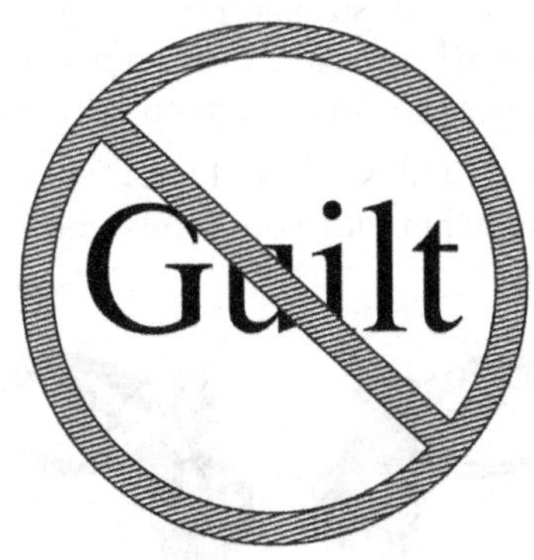

Who needs that?

So, I made a radical lifestyle change. Some people are gluten free; I am guilt free. I am not going to feel guilty about feeling what I feel. Except perhaps feeling guilty that I still feel guilty from time to time (I'm still working on that paradox).

I have given up the self-destructive habit of constant comparison with others. I am going to accept that doing this may be difficult, and that's okay.

I invite you to join me. And if you choose not to, please don't feel guilty. I still love you.

6.

Don't go to the hardware store for milk – in other words, stop repeatedly trying to find something you want or need in the wrong place.

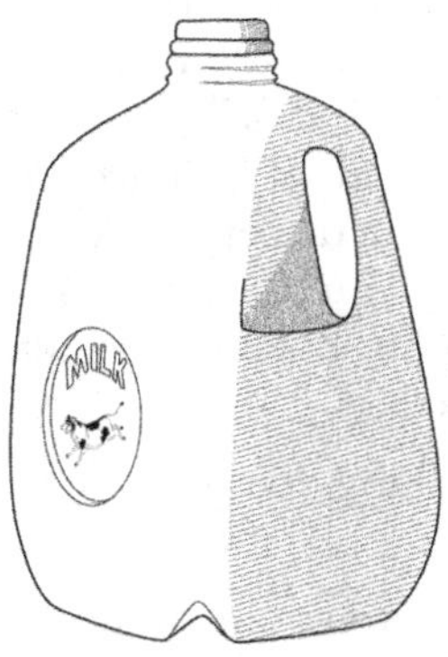

Many of us that struggle with self-destructive habitual thoughts and actions (even though we are otherwise intelligent, insightful, and determined individuals) may find ourselves in similar situations over and over. Despite our intentions, resolve, and misery, there we are again, standing in the (METAPHOR AHEAD) customer service line at the local hardware store, asking the clerk behind the counter where to find the milk. We feel stupid, weak, and hopeless about <u>ever</u> being able to find a way to replace the malignancy of self-loathing with the peacefulness of self-acceptance.

But at the risk of sounding like a hopeless optimist, I fervently believe that deep down inside we are programmed to love ourselves. Beginning a journey of self-acceptance, when you have been accustomed to hating yourself, takes at least some self-love in the first place. The decision to love who you are in this moment (without enrolling in an UBER MAKEOVER BOOT CAMP whose motto is: "IF YOU REALLY LOVED YOURSELF YOU'D LOSE WEIGHT") means that you have a seed of self-acceptance already planted deep inside of you that still loves you. It may be holding on for dear life, but it is there and <u>can</u> be cultivated.

Self-loathing does not start in a vacuum.

If we weren't thrust into a world where all of us were valued for looking a certain way, there would be so many happier people around. There would be fewer women thinking, "I HATE HER," when they see another woman who is thinner or larger breasted or younger than they are. There would be fewer men thinking, "My abs aren't as defined as his, and I don't have as much hair as he does." The competition and jealousy that emerge are divisive because they stem from the formula that aspiring to attain one standard of physical perfection = success = feeling loved and being lovable.

But living in a vacuum is an unrealistic ecosystem, and it would get lonely. We are, for better or worse, living in a society with people (yay!), some of whom, like vacuums, suck (boo).

It would be a lovely respite to live in a safe place where:

- All bodies are considered beautiful and
- Someone may care about what I'm thinking instead of what I look like and,
- We can all dance around naked and not feel ugly or unlovable because of our butts or thighs,

But truthfully, we are living in a world where some people have very negative opinions about how we look. So what to do to start building up our self/size acceptance in this world where size-ism is an accepted form of discrimination and division?

One small step is: Don't go you-know-where for you-know-what!

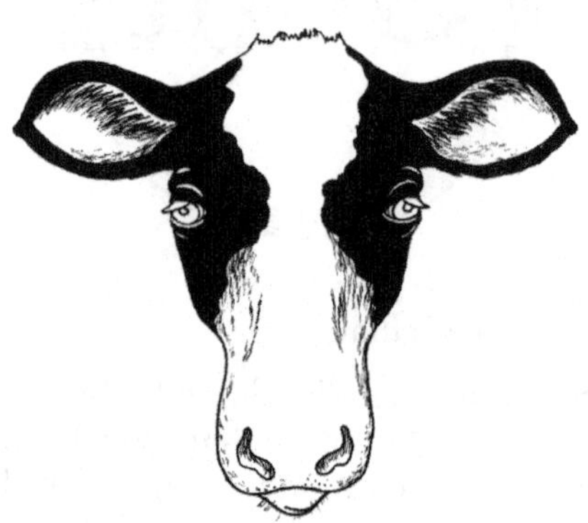

If you go to Thanksgiving Dinner every year knowing people will tell you that you are eating too much, or will comment on your body, and if it feels bad to you and you are shrieking inside your head, "Scotty, beam me up," you are at the hardware store looking for milk.

If you refuse to buy clothing that fits you because you are waiting to be a "normal" size and then sit at home because you have nothing to wear, you are at the hardware store looking for milk.

If you get on the scale every morning and let the number on the scale dictate to you how you will feel that day … get out of the hardware store.

Instead, go to the places that help the self-love inside of you flourish and nourish the seed of self-acceptance.

- Snuggle into the rich soil of friends that have loved you at every size you have been, savor their kindness, and soak in their warmth.
- Get involved in size acceptance and HAES communities.
- Replace negative thoughts with self-affirming thoughts.
- Set limits with people regarding commenting on your size, and if they can't comply, leave. It gets easier with practice – I promise.

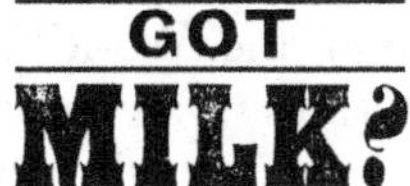

Predictable Challenges

Votes, Veterans, and Vacations. NoVVVember is a month filled with eVents that are emotionally charged for many people. Whether you are political or not, Election Day, especially a presidential election, may stir up controversy amongst friends, colleagues, and family. This time of year we are bombarded by slogans, campaign ads, persuasive friends and family members' opinions urging us to "do the right thing" as Election Day nears. But when we go into that voting booth or face our absentee ballot, we are alone. The choice is all ours. No one has to know what candidates or bond measures we are voting for. We are free to make our own decisions unfettered by external pressure.

This is good advice for living our lives as well. November is not the

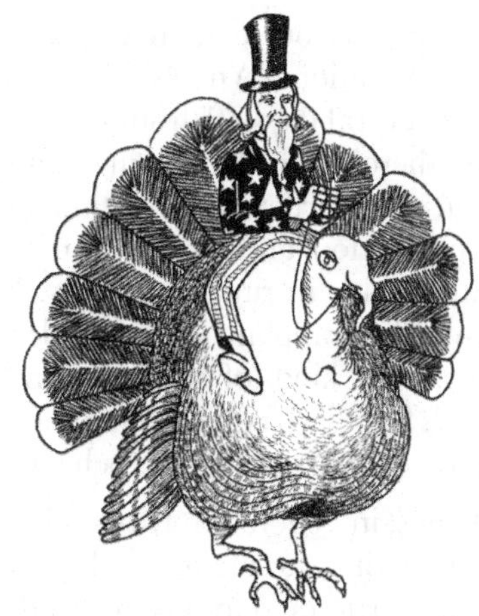

only month when we are flooded with endless messages from the media, loved ones, and colleagues to be the person they want us to be, or to give control over to someone supposedly more competent. When it comes right down to it, it is our choice, every day, how we live our lives, feel about our bodies, manage our stress, and take care of ourselves.

Veteran's Day – especially during years when the country is engaged in military actions and losing service men and women – is a day of mourning and loss. Up until fairly recently, this day was dedicated to wars in our country's past. With fewer people who were old enough to remember the World Wars still alive, Veteran's Day became less meaningful and less of an emotional trigger. Now, however, there are new military actions taking place, and hence, more people are impacted by the real meaning of Veteran's Day.

And then, of course, there is Thanksgiving Vacation. Whether it is one day or several days off from school or work, there is the challenging combination of unstructured free time and the promotion and expectation that we all engage in ritualized feasts. For many folks grappling with disordered eating, these kinds of stressors can be triggers for relapsing and resuming restrictive dieting or bingeing behaviors.

Holidays, in general, may be difficult for many of us to navigate. Because they are promoted and publicized as joyous, happy events, there are many people who do not have that experience. This is so prevalent that there is now term for this: "Holiday Blues."

Depression may worsen if people are feeling disenfranchised from their loved ones or family. Anxiety may increase from the pressure to attend gatherings where there is ambivalence about wanting to participate. Memories of loved ones recently deceased can be sparked that may activate a resurgence of mourning.

And then, of course, there is the food. Thanksgiving is all about the food.

Here are some considerations:

• Overeating is touted as the norm, people are given permission to binge, and this is challenging for clients with eating disorders.

• Family feasts may trigger old habits and behaviors centered on food and body issues.

• The media kicks into gear and elevates the importance and "evil-ness" of food. We are encouraged to indulge and then do "penance for our sins."

• The majority of people struggling with an eating disorder need to prepare for this in advance. If we stay mindful that, although the food is part of the occasion, it isn't THE celebration. We can still listen to our bodies and love who we are, no matter what external messages we are receiving. This is a good time to review ways to manage stress, feelings of sadness, and conflict with others that do not involve using food and/or body hate for self-soothing. Talk about what you are feeling and let people know that not everyone experiences holidays from the same point of view.

Important Dates to Remember

American Diabetes Month – www.diabetes.org
November 11th – Veteran's Day
First Tuesday in November – Election Day
Fourth Thursday in November – Thanksgiving

Proactivity # 1

"ME"lection Day

Materials

Paper, poster board, pencils, markers. Optional: Scissors, glue sticks, magazines.

–

How To

1. Brainstorm and write down at least one upcoming issue that may arise in relation to Election Day, Veteran's Day, Thanksgiving, or any other November-based event – e.g. holiday meals, pressure about dressing up for dinners, political disagreements, loss or absence of a family member in the military, et cetera.

2. Be specific. What is the challenge? Which predicted behaviors are causing anxiety or worry?

3. Now imagine you are a candidate who is campaigning to "fix" these issues. On a separate piece of paper, brainstorm strategies you will put into place when you are "elected" to take care of yourself.

4. Don't censor yourself, but keep the interventions positive and doable. Are there others on your ticket that will reinforce your strategies?

5. Using the art supplies, create a campaign poster with a slogan and at least one specific challenge and action plan the same way a candidate would publicize problems with the economy and promote their plan.

–

Why

The purpose of this directive is to "nominate" ourselves as the person who will best manage the stresses in the November days ahead. This activity helps us to clarify the issues and choices available to tackle them in the best way possible for our health and happiness. It is an opportunity to find our own voice and devise a successful plan.

Notes

Proactivity # 2

Thank-ME Cards

Materials

Card stock paper, markers, pens, pencils, collage materials, glue sticks, postage stamps, and envelopes.

–

How To

1. I know that this may not seem to be the most original of Therapeutic Arts Activities, but because of the unique focus (see "Why" section), it can be a very powerful one.

2. Sit quietly and think about at least one positive contribution that food and/or your body have made in your life.

3. Are there any images, colors, words, which come up that are associated with these positive memories/ connections between food/body and your overall sense of well-being?

4. Using the art materials available, create a thank you card with these images on the outside and then write your appreciation story on the inside. Of course, you can use graphic images on the inside as well – it doesn't need to be just text, as long as it is specific and clear about what is being appreciated and what it is being appreciated for.

5. Put the card inside the self-addressed stamped envelope and either mail it yourself, or, if possible, give the card to someone who will mail it to you. Try to time it so you receive the card close to Thanksgiving.

–

Why

All too often, we focus on the negative aspects of our relationship with food and our bodies and forget that we may have developed some of our attitudes and actions for reasons that – at the time – were the best coping strategies we could come up with. Eventually, we may outgrow these strategies or they may become inappropriate or self- destructive. Intellectually we know they may have outgrown their usefulness, but the integration process takes time. In the meantime, it is important not to vilify yourself for what you have done to take care of yourself the best way you knew how. Thanking your body, fat and all is a healing action. Thanking your food and what it did/does to help you is also a healthy part of the process of change. Writing these notes is a tangible ritual that concretizes this process and allows us to consider options other than self-hate.

Notes

DECEMBER
Ho-Ho-Hope

Personal Perspectives

I know some of us are still basking in the afterglow of Thanksgiving festivities. Good food, good company, and an opportunity to stop and take notice of how much we have to be grateful for. But as we discussed in the last chapter, for some of us, Thanksgiving is more about the battle between the Brillo pad and the crusty burnt residue on the roasting pan than the "happy." Hopefully, however, Thanksgiving was a successful dress rehearsal for the real show that is coming to an emotional theater near you: the winter holidays!

There are many similarities between the two. We may feel obligated to spend time with people we just aren't that crazy about, or we are missing loved ones who are no longer with us. Both occasions force us into situations where the norm is to eat until we are – to grab the obvious metaphor – feeling in solidarity with the other stuffed bird at the table. And because many of us are used to being told that the reason we are fat is because we have no control over our gluttony, we find ourselves thrust into this strange world where we have permission to eat heartily, and may even be coaxed to eat more if we show signs of slowing down. Talk about the opposite of mindful eating! Sure, let's relax and enjoy eating without self-consciousness. What? You are having trouble relaxing? Could it be that relaxing into this parallel universe is out of the question because next on the menu is the expectation that you will join the group ritual of repenting through self-flagellating comments and pledges to NEVER eat again?

For many women, the ordeal starts long before the actual holiday meal. Earlier in the day we have painstakingly wriggled into our Spanx to look as thin as possible. Now we are eating, and paying little attention to our internal cues. Lo and behold- we find the spandex cutting into our bodies like fine cutlery. You'd never know by looking at us that deep crevasses are being formed around our waists that may not fade for days.

Is it any wonder that not everyone LOVES the holidays? Add to the mix several heaping helpings of societal pressure to be happy during the holiday season, and you have a double-edged sword. If a person is feeling anxious, isolated, or depressed, that's difficult enough. But on top of that, there is an added layer of feeling badly for feeling badly. After all, that's not the Holiday Spirit!

Another factor is that the media is pushing us to spend more money than the next person. But honestly, how many of us can afford to give someone a new car? Ask anyone who is struggling with debt, and they will tell you this "present pressure" leads to stress and feelings of inadequacy. But for many, committing the season treason of not over-shopping is unthinkable, and so we pull out the credit cards, light the torch, and let the games begin!

What really irks me is that while fat is decried as being abhorrent in every aspect of our lives, fat is suddenly something to aspire to when describing a person's wallet!

But there is Ho-Ho-Hope.

Not so long ago, we would walk into a Walgreens (or Wal-Mart, etc.) and find only a Christmas aisle. Many of us who did not celebrate Christmas felt marginalized and overlooked for not conforming to the predominant religious "norm." Over the past decade, however, the general public has grown more accepting of the diversity of December celebrations like Kwanzaa, Chanukah, and Winter Solstice, and fewer people feel alienated and overlooked.

As size activists, this is familiar territory.

We know that inclusion and recognition of diversity brings about improved self-esteem and a decrease in feelings of depression and isolation. When we give ourselves and each other permission to feel whatever it is we are feeling during the holidays and to embrace emotional diversity, in addition to size diversity and religious diversity, then making it through December may not be such an Olympic-sized challenge.

As far as the binge shopping goes, let's put away the plastic and splurge on gifts of acceptance, acknowledgment, and support. We won't wind up in debt, and the only interest we will accrue will be interest in each other. I'm guessing that these gifts will last long past the holiday season and, perhaps, all the way into spring training!

Along with the sparkly bangles of Chanukah, Christmas, Kwaanza, Winter Solstice, and New Year's Eve, December is my birthday month. And it also happens to be filled with the birthdays of most of my closest friends! Could there be any astrological meaning to this? I am not talking about my family's birthdays, which are sometimes explained away by certain (ahem) "seasonal" patterns of procreating. I am talking about close friends I have chosen over the years all of whom have birthdays within the same two-week period as my own. Is there a reason why I am drawn to people who are labeled Sagittarians?

Lest you are concerned, please don't worry ... I don't spend an inordinate amount of time thinking about this. I am, after all, a self-proclaimed Astrological Agnostic. I am not certain if that is a bona fide category in the Diagnostic and Statistical Manual of Metaphysics (DSMM) or if I just made up the term. (I know for a fact that there is no such thing as the DSMM, but I have used the Diagnostic and Statistical Manual (DSM) frequently in my professional career, and I have always been tickled by the fact that the word "agnostic" is tidily tucked away inside the word "diagnostic." As a therapist and word junkie I think that is just cool.)

So how do I define an "Astrological Agnostic"?

- Someone who is skeptical about Astrologers' claims that Astrology is an efficacious system of categorizing personalities and predicting possible events in the future;
- Someone who needs statistical proof to eradicate their skepticism about these claims;
- Someone who wouldn't be particularly surprised to find that these claims are legitimate;
- Someone who doesn't judge others who do believe the claims are legitimate.

My cousin writes an Astrology column and is well known for her charts and readings. I find her columns filled with words of wisdom and enjoy reading them, although, being the A.A. that I am, I tend to ignore the Astrological references. I suppose there is a possibility that if she looked at my chart, she would find that the configuration of my planets at the time of my birth is classic for someone who is an Astrological Agnostic. We could set up a study and interview all of the people who have their suns in Sagittarius with Capricorn rising and moons in Aries, et cetera, and ask them to describe their opinion of the validity of Astrological claims. We could then aggregate and analyze the data, accounting for intervening variables and making sure we have a good control group. Then we may find that there is a statistically significant outcome of Astrological Agnostic responses (e.g. "Well, if someone provided me with proof...") associated with those birth charts. These may be data worth noting.

I have no idea. I wasn't planning on talking about Astrology at all, so let's put the zodiac aside and talk about birthday wishes and the moment of wishful blowing (sexual innuendo intendoed). Men and women alike seem to take this traditional candle-blowing, wish-making moment very seriously. I honestly cannot think of a single person who has a nonchalant or laissez-faire candle-blowing approach. Each person pauses, closes their eyes, solemnly reopens them, inhales, and then exhales with the intensity of a dragon or the enthusiasm of an 8-year-old kid. I don't know if making a birthday wish before blowing out the candles is an international tradition, but here are some observations I have made over the years of celebrating birthdays in America:

- Even the most germ-phobic people do not seem to care about the germs and spittle that are being spread over the cake in the process.
- The people waiting for the cake to be served, without any authority figure telling them to be quiet, take on a supportive, silent air in the wish-making pre-candle-blowing moment. (The only exception to this seems to be if someone is documenting this momentous moment with a photo and asks the birthday boy/girl/man/woman to wait a moment so they can prepare the shot.)
- And, of course, the ultimate rule: IF YOU SAY YOUR WISH OUT LOUD, IT WON'T COME TRUE!

This rule is so ingrained in all of us that no one even asks you what you wished for. Well, I am here to tell you that not saying your wish out loud has nothing to do with a wish coming true. If that was the case, I would not have wished the same wish year after year after year. It would have come true and then I would have had the chance to create a new wish each subsequent year. But somehow, during the 364 days that elapsed between opportunities to manifest anything my birthday heart desired, I would forget that it hadn't worked the year before.

Each year I would remind myself not to waste the wish – not to blow it on something superficial and unimportant. After all, it would be another whole year before I would have this much power in my corner. And yet in the final moment … the game-making play … the moment of truth … the birthday genie beckoning … without exception, I would wish…

… to be thin.

Exhale. Done. No take-backs. No do-overs.

Wishing to be thin trumped:

- A new car
- World peace
- Unlimited wealth
- Happy, healthy life
- Happy, healthy kid
- Successful career
- Cure for AIDS

My inner critic always berated me not only for selecting a wish that was primarily about my appearance, but for being totally inconsistent. How could I, an Astrological Agnostic, fervently continue to believe in the magic of birthday wishes despite the preponderance of proof that they did not come true? This pattern continued for decades, until I changed it by giving myself permission to love my body as it is and stop wishing it would be what it wasn't. I still remember the first year I tried my new approach, and wished my son would get into the college of his choice. He did. The next year I wished that a close friend of mine would make it through her fifth year being cancer free. She did! This was a good trend; and no, I don't really believe my wish had anything to do with the outcomes of the two examples I just gave you. After all, correlation is not causation. But, for some inexplicable reason, I feel a twinge of sadness when I think back on all of my birthday wishes wasted. For what? To be thinner waisted? What a waste.

And now, each birthday that I am fortunate enough to celebrate, when I go to blow out the candles on my cake with my loved ones around me, I will have another chance to tap into the magic of the birthday wish.

And while I can't tell you what I will wish for, I bet all of you know what I will not wish for.

The mystery of why most of my chosen friends are Sagittarians continues…

Predictable Challenges

In last month's chapter, we discussed the phenomenon of the "Holiday Blues" and how important it is not to assume that holidays are joyous times for everyone. The month of December continues this trend and is filled with reasons to stay vigilant in this regard. While the beginning of December starts off benign enough, it isn't long before new holiday pressures begin to take center stage. Whether you are a practicing religious person or not, it is difficult to be unaffected by the seductive Sirens of the Winter Holiday Season who are demanding overindulgence in spending, eating, drinking, and partying.

The media promotes the holidays as a time for celebration, indulgence, and conspicuous consumption. This can be a double-edged sword for many who are not feeling particularly jolly – and then feel badly for feeling that way. One way to alleviate this second layer of sadness is by acknowledging the diversity in emotional responses during this season, the same way we have learned to accept diversity in the way different people celebrate the holidays.

The December holidays may be more challenging than Halloween or Thanksgiving. In addition to grappling with the emphasis on holiday feasts, people are encouraged to "binge shop" and express their love through gift giving – sometimes beyond their means. This can be stressful and may trigger old subconscious habits and patterns around eating and body image. Many therapists are on holiday, programs are closed, and this leaves people without their usual support systems, feeling fragile and vulnerable.

Preparing in advance for this challenging time is important, and giving yourself permission to be who you are is vital.

Here are some considerations:

PERMISSION GRANTED: It is okay if you don't feel all HO HO HO during this time of the year. Many of us are going to be reminded of loved ones no longer with us or anniversaries of other events in our lives. Try to accept your feelings and respect your limitations.

PERMISSION GRANTED: It is okay to not go into debt in order to prove that you love your friends and family. Get creative with your gift giving and set a budget you can live with. Honestly, how many of us can really give someone a car with a big red bow as a holiday gift?

PERMISSION GRANTED: Set boundaries with friends and family who want to engage in "diet talk". You can just say no.

PERMISSION GRANTED: Overeating is touted as the norm during the holidays, followed by self-hate and a new resolve to go on a diet on January 1st. You don't have to join in that reindeer game. If it is any consolation, the research shows that most people do not gain inordinate amounts of weight during the holiday season, but the diet industry does gain inordinate amounts of new clients. Try to give yourself the gift of peace of mind. Find ways to diffuse and refuse the pressure to engage in the weight-cycling ritual.

It would be easy to wrap up this month's challenge with the old cliché, "everything in moderation," but that would be misleading. I'm not suggesting that December's therapeutic challenge has to do with maintaining one's "willpower" during Chanukah, Christmas, Kwanzaa, or solstice feasts and celebrations.

I am suggesting that sometimes in the effort to live up to external demands, we get swept away in all of the holiday hoopla and run the risk of losing our connection to our self. When this happens, it is difficult to stop and tune in to the cues our bodies are sending us that we are tired, hungry, full, lonely, or overextended. When we stop listening to our internal signals and needs, we may revert to old habits and may wind up feeling guilty or disappointed in ourselves. For many people, this escalates into an all-or-nothing mindset. Bingeing increases and so does the desperation associated with December 31st, and the compulsion to start all over again with punitive and unrealistic New Year's resolutions.

Some things to consider:

- Practice time management in regard to the upcoming demands of the holiday season, so you don't get overwhelmed by trying to please others while forgetting about self-care.

• Prioritize and budget gift-spending and party-attending so there is a balance between giving to others and not depleting yourself.

• Remember that the holiday season is not joyful for everyone. Be sensitive to those who find this time of year challenging. Try to be honest with yourself and others so you can choose the best way to navigate through the month.

• Whether it is Christmas, Chanukah, Solstice, Kwanzaa, or none of the above, a common theme of this season is supposed to be peace and joy. Find the places (internal or external) of joy and peace that give you strength and reinforce your ability for self-care. Then, set aside some time during the month to spend some time there.

• If you are compelled to set New Year's resolutions, please choose ones that are not based on body hate or numbers on a scale. Set short-term, attainable goals that are more related to self-acceptance.

Important Dates to Remember

December 21st – Winter Solstice
December 25 – Christmas
December 26-January 1 – Kwanzaa
Chanukah – Varies but is usually within the first three weeks of December

Proactivity # 1

Permission Slips

Materials

Lined paper, unlined drawing paper, pencils, markers, collage materials, glue sticks.

—

How To

1. Take a moment to sit quietly and identify one triggering expectation that you will face during the upcoming holiday season. It can be about food, body image, pleasing a relative, gift giving, etc. It can be a scenario that you have already lived through or one you predict will arise in the upcoming weeks.

2. Write down the scenario in as much detail as possible. Make sure the scenario contains a beginning, middle, and end of the event, a list of the people involved, and the location(s) of the event.

3. Identify one point in the scenario where having permission to do or say something differently may result in a positive change to the scenario. On a separate piece of paper, write down the new version.

4. Using the art supplies, create a personal permission slip. This can take any form you want, as long as there is a line for a signature.

5. Sign the permission slip and keep it in a place where you can check in with it from time to time during the month.

–

Why

The holiday season is frequently about pleasing others and grappling with the enormous pressure to conform to societal standards around food, appearance, and expressions of love. Suppressing feelings can trigger disordered eating, and holiday stress can result in falling back on default modes of self-hate and feelings of not being good enough. This directive provides the opportunity to anticipate challenges and plan a problem solving strategy. The goal is that if you find yourself in these situations in real life, you will be able to tackle them with increased awareness and a stronger internal support mechanism.

Notes

Notes

Proactivity # 2

S(elf) Help Coupons

Materials

Paper (either plain white drawing or multi-color construction), markers, pens, scissors, glue sticks, magazines.

–

How to

1. Brainstorm on one to four realistic ways to find a place of peace or source of joy to tap into during the month of December. This can be as simple as sitting quietly somewhere, listening to a favorite CD, doing a crossword puzzle, going to a museum, or unplugging your phone for an hour. Whatever you choose, remember that the purpose is to have an opportunity to check in with your thoughts and needs, and to replenish yourself.

2. Using the model of a coupon or gift card, put one idea on each piece of paper using symbols, pictures, words, colors, et cetera. Go all out, as if it is a gift you are giving someone else, because we frequently put more effort into contributing to the happiness of other people than we do ourselves. This coupon is a gift-note to yourself to remind you to take some self-care time.

3. You can put the coupons in gift boxes or envelopes and open them periodically during the holiday season. If you have a friend or relative who will "play along," have them give you the gifts or hide them around your home for you to find during the month.

–

Why

The winter holiday season – when stripped of the emphasis on commercialism and overindulgence – is, at its core, about joy, peace, and the changing of the season. Remembering to focus on those aspects during the month of December is truly helpful if we want to stay connected to the inner cues our body is sending us. This expressive arts therapy directive is a playful way to remember how not to lose ourselves while we are engaged in the whirlwind of giving to others. Remember: If you are unable to follow through with the suggestions on the cards, please do not punish yourself. Take a moment and consider what barriers kept you from following through on these self-care activities. Sometimes the reason why we don't do something is valuable information that will help us make changes in the future.

Notes

THE CELERY CONNECTION

INCH BY INCH, ROW BY ROW, I'M GONNA MAKE MY GARDEN GROW.

– DAVID MALLETT

We moved from Queens to Long Island in order to live in a neighborhood with a better school district. Walking into the classroom that first morning, I knew immediately that this was better. Unlike my former inner city school, the room was filled with books, science equipment, clean desks, posters, and a greenhouse window. It was the greenhouse that caught my eye. There was a row of celery stalks each one a different color; magenta, blue, black, violet and the original green. There was also one stalk that was, to me, a repulsive color resembling puke and mayonnaise. How had Mrs. Markowitz, my new third grade teacher, turned the celery into such a rainbow of colors? It turned out it wasn't quite as magical as I had imagined. Later in the week she explained that if we put food coloring in the soil it seeped into the celery and transformed it into a totally different looking stalk. Underneath the new colorful façade, the celery remained mostly unchanged.

–

What was different was the way it was viewed by others. We liked the prettier celery more and fought over who would get to take the purple one home! The "pukey" stalk was rejected because it was ugly and the plain green celery stalk was ignored because it was so boring. Mrs. M. patiently explained that the green celery was actually healthier for us to eat because it had no food coloring. It was brilliant the way she took that lesson and showed us how we can influence living things by the way we take care of them. Sometimes the impact is superficial and not harmful and other times it can be destructive and irreversible. And most importantly, she pointed out, people are not always making a good choice by opting for something based on its beauty factor.

–

Of course Mrs. Markowitz had no idea that she was teaching a lesson about weight stigma and body hate.

I didn't know it either until much later in my life when I made the "Celery Connection".

–

All of the years of teasing and rejection because of other people's judgments about my body defined me for a large part of my life. And despite a long list of accomplishments, I felt un-loveable and alone. My soil had been tainted with toxic elements of criticism about my body. I was being fertilized with negative messages about my weight and irrigated with warnings that I was unacceptable. I embodied the messages and they spread through me leaving me feeling like the "pukey" mayo celery stalk. But deep inside me were the seeds of thought planted all those years ago in Mrs. M's class. Seeds that taught me that people should not love me less because of what I looked like. It's not that I wanted to be loved <u>because</u> I was fat, I just didn't want to be un-loved <u>because</u> I was fat. I also didn't want to be loved <u>because</u> I was thin. What I really wanted was to love myself for who I was naturally; a curvy, short, red-haired, and outspoken "stalk of celery".

–

And that is who has written this book. I know that not everyone will love me and/or love my body. I have no power over what <u>everyone</u> thinks. I have power over what I think and I am no longer waiting to live my life or love my body. Now <u>that</u> is a garden worth tending and cultivating.

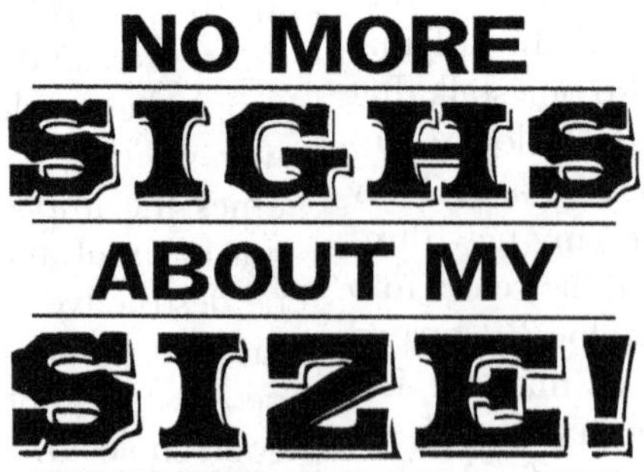

WHAT'S GROWIN' ON?

30 days hath September, April, June, and November… Now that we have spent the year together (how time does fly!) I am hoping that I was able to effectively communicate how each month has elements of consistency and elements of change. Each month provides us with opportunities for building self-awareness, growing self-acceptance, and learning more about how to accept the natural diversity of our bodies, and not to give others the power to foster self-hate.

—

It has been a privilege to share some of what I have learned from my personal and professional experiences with body image and disordered eating, and I hope that my musings have been helpful in some way with your own journey. If you would like to drop me a line and let me know, feel free to contact me at **drdeah@drdeah.com**.

MAY YOUR

SELF-ACCEPTANCE

AND

BODY IMAGE

FLOURISH!

RESOURCES

I have been professionally involved in the field of Size Acceptance, eating disorders, and body image since the 1980s and personally involved since childhood. The fact that there is still so much work to do to help prevent eating disorders and battle the discrimination and bullying towards any population that does not fit into society's standards for beauty, can be discouraging at times. What I do find hopeful, however, is that the list of people working in the field of Health at Every Size (HAES) and Size Acceptance is growing.

–

Community is vital. For those of us fighting to change our personal standards of beauty and self-worth, the support we can give each other by sharing resources is enormously important. Here are some Professional Organizations that I would like to share with you. Although this book will not be updated frequently, the resource list on my website is constantly growing and includes books, blogs, treatment programs, and clinicians. Come visit the website and if you have a resource you think I should add, please email the information to **drdeah@drdeah.com** and I will include them. Please remember though, this is not a resource list for diet books or weight loss methods and I don't receive any financial compensations from the people and organizations on the list.

–

Size Acceptance and Eating Disorders Professional Organizations

Association of Anorexia Nervosa and Associated Disorders (ANAD)
ANAD.ORG

Association for Professionals Treating Eating Disorders (APTED)
APTEDSF.COM

Association of Size Diversity and Health (ASDAH)
SIZEDIVERSITYANDHEALTH.ORG

Binge Eating Disorder Association (BEDA)
BEDAONLINE.COM

Education and Therapy for Eating Disorders (EATFED)
FACEBOOK.COM/PAGES/EATFED-EDUCATION-AND-THERAPY-FOR-EATING-DISORDERS/195759940466862

National Association to Advance Fat Acceptance (NAAFA)
NAAFA.ORG

National Eating Disorders Association (NEDA)
NATIONALEATINGDISORDERS.ORG

Expressive Arts and Recreation Therapy Professional Organizations

American Art Therapy Association (AATA)
ARTTHERAPY.ORG

American Dance Therapy Association (ADTA)
ADTA.ORG

American Music Therapy Association (AMTA)
MUSICTHERAPY.ORG

American Society of Group Psychotherapy and Psychodrama (ASGPP)
ASGPP.ORG

American Therapeutic Recreation Association (ATRA)
ATRA-ONLINE.COM

International Expressive Arts Therapy Association (IEATA)
IEATA.ORG

Mental Fitness Inc. (formerly NORMAL in the Schools), a non-profit organization providing school programs in body image.
MENTALFITNESSINC.ORG

National Association of Drama Therapy (NADT)
NADT.ORG

National Association for Poetry Therapy (NAPT)
POETRYTHERAPY.ORG

National Coalition of Creative Arts Therapies Associations (NCCATA)
NCCATA.ORG

ABOUT THE AUTHOR

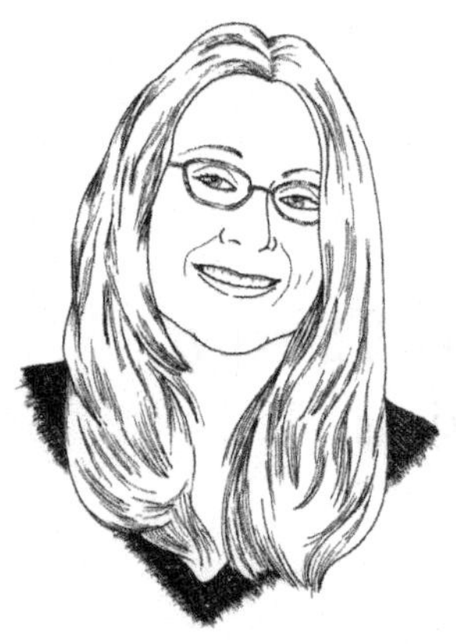

DR. DEAH SCHWARTZ, EDUCATOR, CLINICIAN, ACTIVIST, AND AUTHOR, has extensive experience employing expressive arts therapy to treat eating disorders and body image dissatisfaction. Dr. Deah's private practice in Oakland, California (Dr. Deah's Walkie Talkies), is comprised of sessions specifically tailored for clients who feel as if they do not have enough time in their schedule to fit in healthy movement and verbal therapy. In Dr. Deah's sessions, she walks with her clients as they discuss their body image issues and disordered eating patterns. At the end of the session, the client can cross two things off of his or her "To Do" list. One of the goals of these sessions is to introduce the client to local trails and other opportunities for pleasurable physical activity NOT associated with weight loss. If you are interested in training so you can incorporate Walkie Talkie sessions into your practice, or want to book sessions with Dr. Deah, contact her at **drdeah@drdeah.com**.

Deah is the co-author of *Leftovers: The Ups and Downs of a Compulsive Eater* DVD/Workbook Set, a resource for eating disorders and body dissatisfaction that includes the DVD of the Off-Broadway play, *Leftovers: The Ups and Downs of a Compulsive Eater*. Dr. Schwartz, a member of Actor's Equity, is also one of three actresses that co-starred and co-wrote the play. The DVD/workbook set and DVD are for sale on Dr. Deah's Body Shop website at **drdeah.com**.

Dr. Deah's syndicated blog, *Tasty Morsels*, can be found on her website, and on the following size acceptance, eating disorders, and expressive arts websites:

Adios Barbie

Art Therapy Blog

ASDAH HAES Files

BEDA Weight Stigma Week Campaign

Curvy Lingerie Love Your Body Campaign

Eating Disorders On Line

Eating Disorders Resource Center

Fierce Freethinking Fatties

More of Me to Love

National Eating Disorders Association

Peresephone Magazine

We are the Real Deal

—

Her writing is included in the following publications:

Breaking the Bonds of Food Addiction by Susan McQuillan

Hot and Heavy: Fierce Fat Girls on Life, Love, and Fashion, edited by Virgie Tovar

Therapy Techniques: Using the Creative Arts by Ann Arge Nathan

Fat Poets Speak: Living and Loving Fatly, edited by Frannie Zellman

The Politics of Size: Perspectives from the Fat-acceptance Movement, edited by Ragen Chastain

—

Dr. Schwartz is a trainer using the Health for Every Body Curriculum developed by Laura McKibben and Dr. Jon Robison for professional corporate wellness programs and was on the team that reviewed the collaborative efforts of NAAFA, ASDAH, and SNEB's Health at Every Size curriculum.

Deah is available for speaking engagements and has presented at professional organization conferences which include:

American Society of Group Psychotherapy and Psychodrama

Association for Size Diversity and Health

American Therapeutic Recreation Association

Bay Area Social Workers in Healthcare

Binge Eating Disorders Association

Expressive Therapies Summit

National Association to Advance Fat Acceptance

Petaluma Eating Disorders Dieticians

Popular Culture Association

—

To find out more about Dr. Deah's work, visit her website at **drdeah.com** or contact her at **drdeah@drdeah.com**

CPSIA information can be obtained at www.ICGtesting.com
Printed in the USA
LVOW04s1424250215

428307LV00005B/316/P